Mthfr Cookbook

For Fertility

Optimizing Your Nutrition, Food Choices, and Genetics for Delicious Recipes

DR JANE T. RYAN

INTRODUCTION

 Welcome to the tantalizing world of the MTHFR Cookbook for Fertility, where the art of crafting delectable dishes meets the science of supporting reproductive wellness. Unleash a symphony of flavors that not only excite your taste buds but also cater to the unique needs of individuals navigating the intricate path of fertility. From zesty recipes designed to ignite your palate to the carefully curated ingredients that dance harmoniously with MTHFR considerations, this cookbook is your passport to a spicy culinary journey that embraces both health and indulgence. Let the vibrant fusion of spices and fertility-friendly goodness transform your kitchen into a haven of savory delights, setting the stage for a flavorful exploration of nourishing your body and nurturing your fertility. Get ready to embark on a gastronomic adventure where every bite is a step toward wellness, spiced just right for your fertility journey.

Understanding Mthfr And Its Impact On Fertility

Delve into the intricate realm of MTHFR and its profound influence on fertility as we unravel the connection within the pages of the MTHFR Cookbook for Fertility. Begin by demystifying the MTHFR gene variant, understanding its role in methylation processes crucial for overall health and reproductive well-being.

Embark on a journey through insightful content that elucidates how MTHFR variations may impact fertility, exploring the potential links to recurrent pregnancy loss, implantation issues, and hormonal imbalances. Navigate the scientific nuances with clarity, empowering readers with knowledge to make informed dietary choices tailored to their specific genetic landscape.

This cookbook isn't just a collection of recipes; it's a guide that harmonizes the culinary arts with fertility science. Discover nutrient-dense ingredients and spice combinations strategically chosen to complement MTHFR considerations, fostering an environment conducive to optimal reproductive health. From fertility-boosting superfoods to mouthwatering dishes designed to support methylation pathways, each recipe is a flavorful step towards enhancing fertility.

Dive into a comprehensive exploration of the MTHFR Cookbook, where understanding the genetic puzzle of fertility meets the artistry of creating meals that are both health-conscious and delectable. Let this resource be your companion on the path to embracing the science of MTHFR while savoring the richness of flavors that contribute to your fertility journey.

Importance Of Nutrition For Fertility

Embark on a culinary voyage with the MTHFR Cookbook for Fertility, where the significance of nutrition takes center stage in the quest for optimal reproductive health. Delving into the importance of nutrition for fertility, this comprehensive guide elucidates how the right balance of nutrients can create a conducive environment for conception.

Explore the profound impact of specific nutrients on hormonal balance, egg quality, and sperm health. From the crucial role of antioxidants in combating oxidative stress to the influence of vitamins and minerals on reproductive function, every aspect of nutrition is meticulously addressed.

This cookbook transforms the kitchen into a laboratory of fertility-boosting concoctions, emphasizing the role of nutrient-dense ingredients in supporting methylation processes. Discover the power of omega-3 fatty acids, folate-rich foods, and fertility-enhancing herbs meticulously woven into recipes that not only nourish the body but also cater to the unique needs of those with MTHFR variations.

Navigate the complexities of fertility nutrition with ease, as this cookbook bridges the gap between scientific understanding and practical application. From preconception to pregnancy, each recipe is crafted to harness the benefits of specific nutrients, creating a symphony of flavors that align with the principles of fertility science.

Elevate your culinary experience with the MTHFR Cookbook for Fertility, where nutrition becomes a delicious ally on the journey to conception. Let this guide be your compass, navigating the landscape of fertility with a palette of flavors that not only tantalize the taste buds but also contribute to the holistic well-being of individuals striving to enhance their fertility through the power of nutrition.

CHAPTER 1

MTHFR BASICS

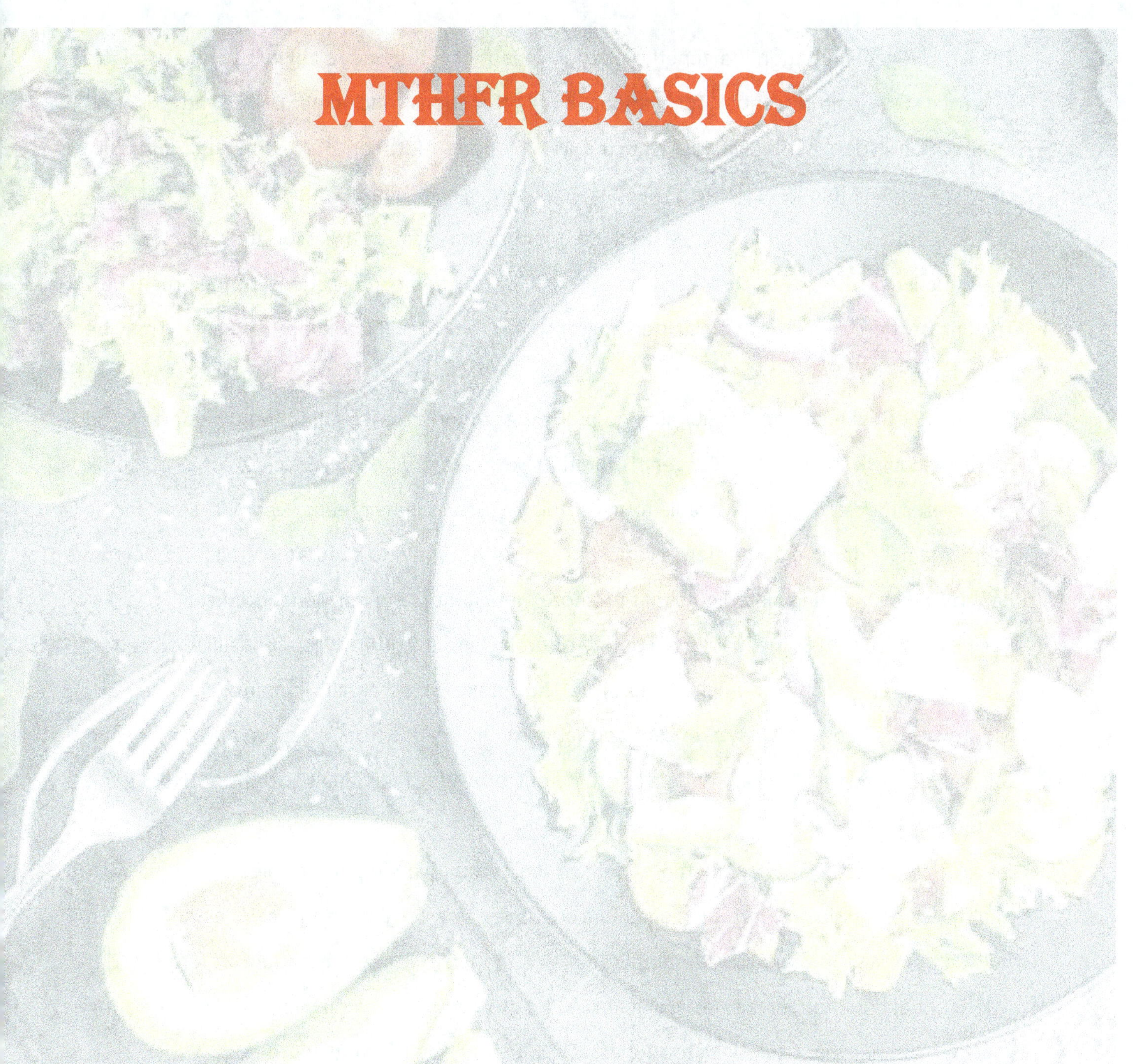

OVERVIEW OF MTHFR GENE MUTATION

The MTHFR gene mutation is a genetic variation that affects the body's ability to process folate, a crucial B-vitamin essential for various bodily functions, including DNA synthesis and methylation processes. Individuals with the MTHFR gene mutation may experience difficulty converting folate into its active form, leading to potential health implications.

In the context of fertility, the MTHFR gene mutation has been associated with certain reproductive challenges, such as recurrent pregnancy loss and complications during pregnancy. To address these concerns, a specialized approach like the MTHFR Cookbook for Fertility may be considered.

The MTHFR Cookbook for Fertility aims to provide a comprehensive guide to nutrition tailored for individuals with the MTHFR gene mutation who are trying to conceive. The cookbook emphasizes foods rich in bioavailable forms of folate, such as leafy greens, legumes, and specific supplements. Additionally, it offers a variety of recipes designed to support overall reproductive health by incorporating ingredients that promote methylation and hormonal balance.

Recipes in the MTHFR Cookbook for Fertility often include nutrient-dense foods like avocados, eggs, and lean proteins, aiming to optimize the intake of essential vitamins and minerals. Moreover, the cookbook may provide information on lifestyle factors, stress management, and other considerations that can influence fertility outcomes for individuals with the MTHFR gene mutation.

It's crucial to note that while dietary modifications can play a supportive role, consulting with healthcare professionals, including a genetic counselor or a fertility specialist, is essential for a holistic approach to managing the implications of the MTHFR gene mutation on fertility. The MTHFR Cookbook for Fertility serves as a resource to complement medical guidance, offering practical and nutritious solutions to support individuals on their fertility journey.

How MTHFR Affects Fertility

The MTHFR gene mutation can impact fertility by influencing various biological processes essential for reproductive health. This genetic variation can affect the body's ability to convert folate into its active form, leading to potential complications that may impact fertility. Here's an in-depth look at how MTHFR affects fertility and the role of the MTHFR Cookbook for Fertility in addressing these concerns:

1. Methylation Process:

- The MTHFR gene is involved in the methylation process, a crucial biochemical reaction responsible for DNA synthesis, repair, and regulation of gene expression.
- A mutated MTHFR gene may result in reduced efficiency in methylation, potentially affecting the regulation of genes involved in fertility and reproductive processes.

2. Folate Metabolism:

- Folate is vital for the development of a healthy fetus and plays a key role in preventing neural tube defects.
- MTHFR gene mutation can hinder the conversion of folate into its active form (5-MTHF), leading to decreased availability of this essential nutrient for crucial processes during early pregnancy.

3. Increased Homocysteine Levels:

- The MTHFR mutation can elevate homocysteine levels in the blood, which is associated with adverse pregnancy outcomes, including recurrent miscarriages and preeclampsia.
- Elevated homocysteine levels may contribute to impaired blood flow to the uterus, potentially affecting implantation and fetal development.

4. Impact on Hormonal Balance:

- Methylation processes influenced by MTHFR can impact hormonal balance, including estrogen metabolism.

- Hormonal imbalances may affect the menstrual cycle, ovulation, and overall reproductive function.

5. Role of MTHFR Cookbook for Fertility:

- The MTHFR Cookbook for Fertility is designed to address these concerns by providing targeted nutritional guidance.
- Recipes in the cookbook focus on foods rich in bioavailable forms of folate, supporting individuals with the MTHFR gene mutation in obtaining essential nutrients for reproductive health.

6. Nutrient-Dense Recipes:

- The cookbook includes recipes incorporating nutrient-dense foods known to support fertility, such as leafy greens, avocados, eggs, and lean proteins.
- By emphasizing specific ingredients, the cookbook aims to optimize nutrient intake and promote a healthy environment for conception.

7. Comprehensive Approach:

- While the MTHFR Cookbook for Fertility is a valuable resource, it's essential to complement dietary changes with medical guidance.
- Consultation with healthcare professionals, including genetic counselors and fertility specialists, is crucial to tailor an individualized approach considering the broader aspects of fertility.

understanding how the MTHFR gene mutation affects fertility provides the basis for targeted interventions, and the MTHFR Cookbook for Fertility serves as a supportive tool by offering practical dietary solutions to enhance reproductive health in individuals with this genetic variation.

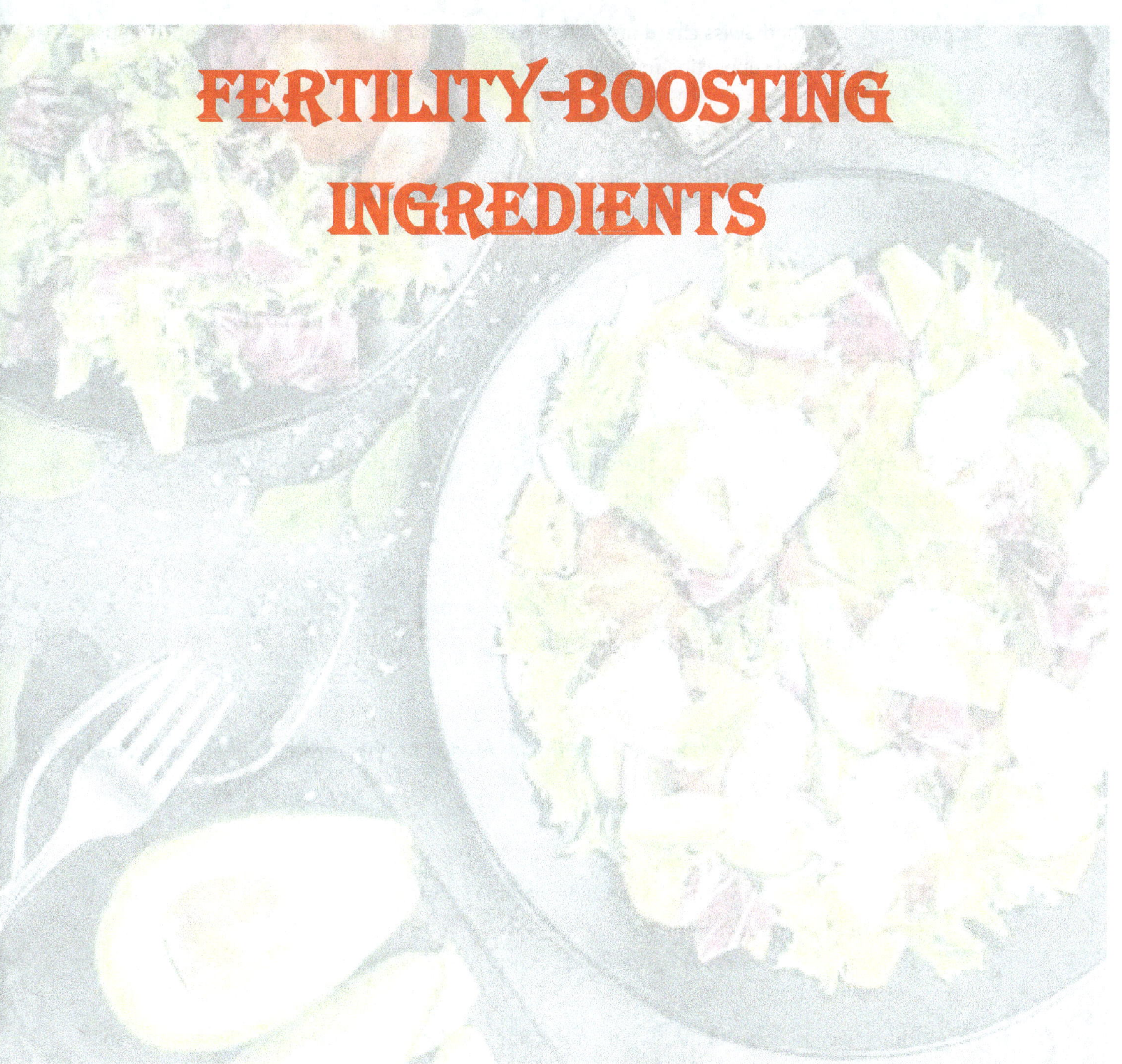

CHAPTER 2

FERTILITY-BOOSTING INGREDIENTS

LIST OF NUTRIENT-RICH FOODS

Leafy Greens:

- Spinach, kale, and Swiss chard are rich in folate, a crucial nutrient for preventing neural tube defects and supporting fertility.

Berries:

- Blueberries, strawberries, and raspberries contain antioxidants that may help improve egg quality and reduce oxidative stress.

Avocado:

- Packed with monounsaturated fats, avocados support hormone production, including those essential for fertility.

Fatty Fish:

- Salmon, mackerel, and trout are high in omega-3 fatty acids, which play a role in reproductive health and may enhance fertility.

Nuts and Seeds:

- Walnuts, almonds, flaxseeds, and chia seeds provide essential fatty acids, zinc, and selenium, promoting reproductive health.

Legumes:

- Lentils, chickpeas, and black beans offer a good source of protein, fiber, and folate, supporting overall fertility.

Whole Grains:

- Quinoa, brown rice, and oats provide complex carbohydrates, fiber, and B vitamins, essential for reproductive health.

Dairy or Dairy Alternatives:

- Rich in calcium and vitamin D, dairy products and fortified alternatives like almond milk contribute to reproductive well-being.

Eggs:

- Eggs are a complete protein source and contain choline, which is crucial for fetal brain development.

Lean Protein:

- Chicken, turkey, and lean beef offer high-quality protein, iron, and zinc, supporting fertility and reproductive function.

Citrus Fruits:

- Oranges, grapefruits, and lemons provide vitamin C, which may enhance sperm quality and reduce the risk of ovulatory disorders.

Sweet Potatoes:

- Rich in beta-carotene, sweet potatoes support overall reproductive health and may improve fertility.

Broccoli:

- A powerhouse of nutrients, including vitamins C and K, folate, and fiber, broccoli supports hormonal balance.

Pomegranate:

- Known for its antioxidant properties, pomegranate may improve blood flow to the uterus and enhance fertility.

Dark Chocolate:

- High-quality dark chocolate in moderation provides antioxidants and may positively impact fertility by reducing stress.
- Remember, a balanced and varied diet, combined with a healthy lifestyle, can contribute to overall fertility and reproductive well-being. It's advisable to consult with a healthcare professional or a nutritionist for personalized advice based on individual health conditions.

IMPORTANCE OF ORGANIC AND WHOLE FOODS

- Certainly, the importance of organic and whole foods in the context of fertility can be significant. Here's a detailed look at how these types of foods can contribute to fertility-boosting ingredients:

Reduced Pesticide Exposure:

- Organic Foods: Choosing organic fruits, vegetables, and grains can minimize exposure to synthetic pesticides and herbicides. Pesticides may interfere with hormonal balance, and reducing their intake could be beneficial for reproductive health.

Nutrient Density:

- Whole Foods: Whole foods, including fruits, vegetables, whole grains, and lean proteins, are rich in essential nutrients. These nutrients, such as vitamins, minerals, and antioxidants, play a crucial role in reproductive health, supporting both male and female fertility.

Balanced Hormones:

- Organic Meats: Opting for organic and grass-fed meats can provide a healthier balance of omega-3 and omega-6 fatty acids. This balance is essential for hormonal regulation, which influences reproductive function.

Preservation of Nutrients:

- Whole Foods: Processing and refining can strip foods of their natural nutrients. Whole foods retain their original nutritional composition, ensuring that the body receives a broad spectrum of essential nutrients required for optimal fertility.

Avoiding Hormone Disruptors:

- Organic Dairy: Choosing organic dairy products helps avoid the potential intake of synthetic hormones and antibiotics. Hormone disruptors in conventional dairy could impact reproductive hormones and fertility.

Improved Digestive Health:

- Whole Grains and Fiber-Rich Foods: Whole grains and fiber support healthy digestion and help regulate blood sugar levels. Stable blood sugar is crucial for hormonal balance, positively influencing fertility.

Omega-3 Fatty Acids:

- Organic and Wild-Caught Fish: Opting for organic and wild-caught fish as sources of omega-3 fatty acids can contribute to reducing inflammation and supporting reproductive health.

Antioxidant Protection:

- Organic Fruits and Vegetables: Organic produce tends to have higher levels of antioxidants. Antioxidants protect the body from oxidative stress, which can negatively impact fertility by damaging reproductive cells.

Glyphosate Avoidance:

- Organic Foods: Glyphosate, a common herbicide, has been associated with potential reproductive issues. Choosing organic foods can help minimize exposure to glyphosate.

Alkaline Balance:

- Whole Plant-Based Foods: A diet rich in whole, plant-based foods contributes to an alkaline environment in the body. Some studies suggest that an alkaline pH may support fertility.
- It's important to note that while choosing organic and whole foods can be beneficial for fertility, an overall balanced and varied diet, along with a healthy lifestyle, is crucial. Consulting with healthcare professionals or nutritionists for personalized advice based on individual health conditions is recommended.

CHAPTER 3

MEAL PLANNING FOR FERTILITY

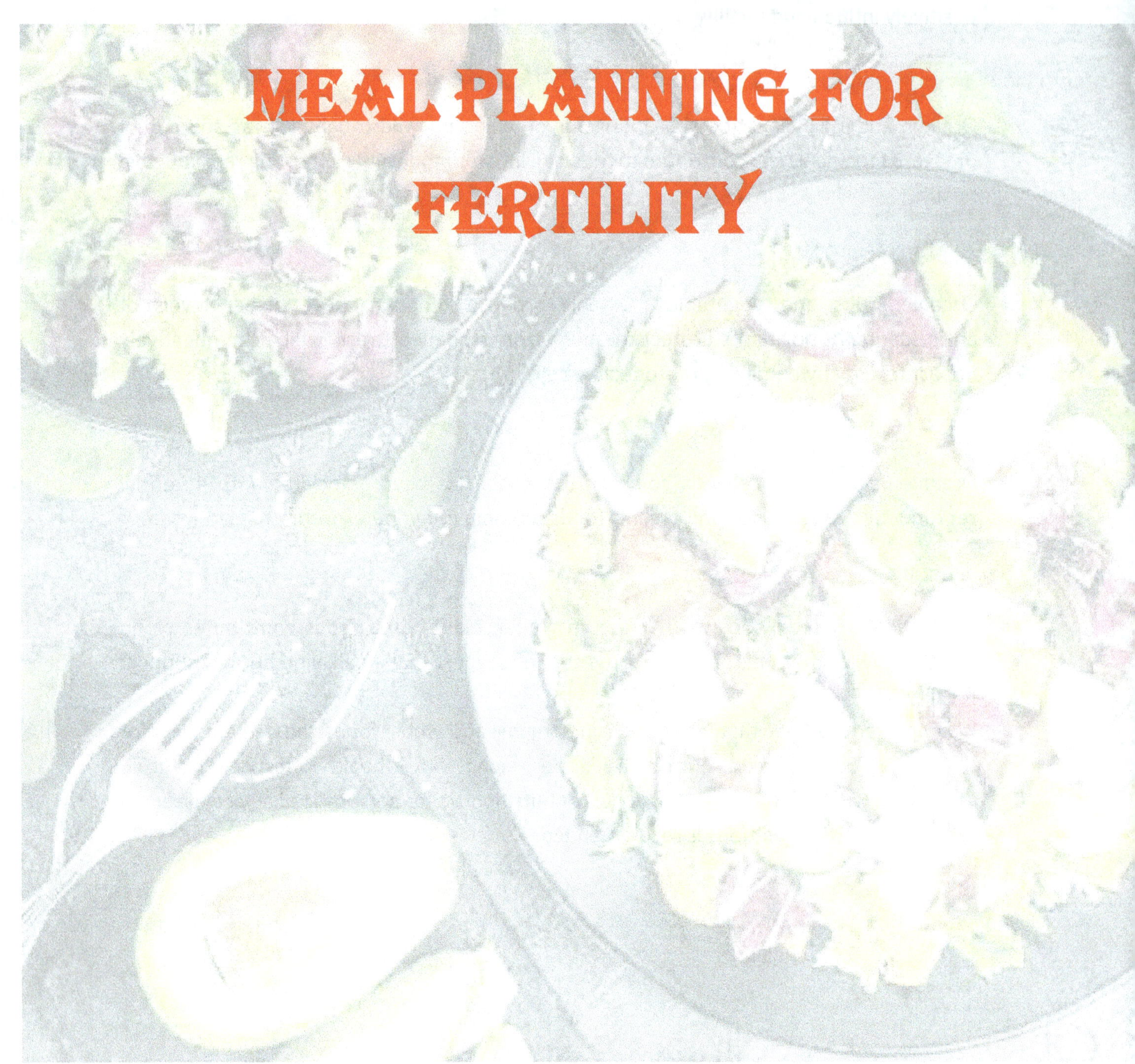

Building A Balanced Fertility Diet

- Building a balanced fertility diet through thoughtful meal planning is crucial for optimizing reproductive health. Consider incorporating the following elements into your meals:

Macronutrients:

Protein:

- Include lean sources such as poultry, fish, beans, and tofu. Protein is essential for cell growth and repair.

Carbohydrates:

- Choose complex carbs like whole grains, fruits, and vegetables. They provide sustained energy and regulate blood sugar levels.

Healthy Fats:

- Opt for sources like avocados, nuts, and olive oil. These fats support hormone production critical for fertility.

Micronutrients:

Folate:

- Found in leafy greens, legumes, and citrus fruits, folate is crucial for preventing neural tube defects in early pregnancy.

Iron:

- Incorporate iron-rich foods like lean meats, beans, and spinach to support healthy blood flow, which is vital for fertility.

Zinc:

- Seeds, nuts, and dairy products are good sources of zinc, a mineral essential for reproductive health and DNA synthesis.

Vitamins C and E:

- These antioxidants, present in fruits and vegetables, can protect eggs and sperm from oxidative stress.

Omega-3 Fatty Acids:

- Include fatty fish like salmon, chia seeds, and walnuts for their omega-3 fatty acids. These support hormonal balance and may improve egg quality.

Hydration:

- Stay well-hydrated with water and herbal teas. Proper hydration helps maintain cervical mucus consistency, crucial for sperm motility.

Limit Processed Foods:

- Minimize processed foods, as they often contain added sugars and unhealthy fats. These can disrupt hormonal balance and impact fertility.

Moderate Caffeine and Alcohol:

- Limit caffeine intake and alcohol consumption, as excessive amounts can affect fertility. Opt for herbal teas or decaffeinated options.

Regular Meals:

- Aim for regular, balanced meals to maintain stable blood sugar levels. This can positively influence hormone regulation and reproductive health.

Include Dairy or Alternatives:

- Ensure an adequate intake of calcium, which is crucial for bone health. Choose low-fat dairy or fortified plant-based alternatives.

Mindful Eating:

- Practice mindful eating to foster a healthy relationship with food. Stress management is vital for fertility, and mindful eating can contribute to overall well-being.

Consult with a Nutritionist or Healthcare Professional:

- Individual needs vary, and consulting with a nutritionist or healthcare professional can provide personalized guidance based on specific fertility concerns.
- Remember, a balanced fertility diet is part of an overall healthy lifestyle. Combine it with regular exercise, stress management, and sufficient sleep for comprehensive reproductive well-being.

4 Weeks Sample Meal Plans

Week 1:

Day 1:

- Breakfast: MTHFR-Friendly Smoothie Bowl
- Lunch: Lentil and Vegetable Wrap
- Dinner: Baked Salmon with Lemon and Dill

Day 2:

- Breakfast: Quinoa and Vegetable Breakfast Bowl
- Lunch: Sweet Potato and Chickpea Buddha Bowl
- Dinner: Quinoa-Stuffed Bell Peppers

Day 3:

- Breakfast: Avocado and Spinach Omelette
- Lunch: Salmon and Avocado Salad
- Dinner: Turmeric Chicken Stir-Fry

Day 4:

- Breakfast: Greek Yogurt Parfait with Berries
- Lunch: Nut and Seed Trail Mix
- Dinner: Roasted Brussels Sprouts with Garlic

Week 2:

Day 1:

- Breakfast: Almond and Chia Seed Energy Bites
- Lunch: Lentil and Vegetable Wrap
- Dinner: Quinoa-Stuffed Bell Peppers

Day 2:

- Breakfast: MTHFR-Friendly Smoothie Bowl
- Lunch: Sweet Potato and Chickpea Buddha Bowl
- Dinner: Baked Salmon with Lemon and Dill

- Breakfast: Greek Yogurt Parfait with Berries
- Lunch: Turmeric Chicken Stir-Fry
- Dinner: Cauliflower Mash

Day 4:

- Breakfast: Chia Seed Pudding with Mango
- Lunch: Salmon and Avocado Salad
- Dinner: Ginger and Turmeric Infused Water

Week 3:

Day 1:

- Breakfast: Avocado and Spinach Omelet
- Lunch: Nut and Seed Trail Mix
- Dinner: Roasted Brussels Sprouts with Garlic

Day 2:

- Breakfast: Quinoa and Vegetable Breakfast Bowl
- Lunch: Lentil and Vegetable Wrap
- Dinner: Turmeric Chicken Stir-Fry

Day 3:

- Breakfast: Greek Yogurt Parfait with Berries
- Lunch: Sweet Potato and Chickpea Buddha Bowl
- Dinner: Baked Salmon with Lemon and Dill

Day 4:

- Breakfast: MTHFR-Friendly Smoothie Bowl
- Lunch: Quinoa-Stuffed Bell Peppers
- Dinner: Cauliflower Mash

Week 4:

Day 1:

- Breakfast: Almond and Chia Seed Energy Bites
- Lunch: Salmon and Avocado Salad

- Dinner: Ginger and Turmeric Infused Water

- Breakfast: Chia Seed Pudding with Mango
- Lunch: Lentil and Vegetable Wrap
- Dinner: Quinoa-Stuffed Bell Peppers

- Breakfast: Avocado and Spinach Omelet
- Lunch: Sweet Potato and Chickpea Buddha Bowl
- Dinner: Roasted Brussels Sprouts with Garlic

- Breakfast: MTHFR-Friendly Smoothie Bowl
- Lunch: Nut and Seed Trail Mix
- Dinner: Baked Salmon with Lemon and Dill

Feel free to adjust portion sizes based on individual needs and preferences. It's essential to stay hydrated throughout the day and consider any specific dietary requirements or restrictions.

CHAPTER 4

RECIPES FOR BREAKFAST

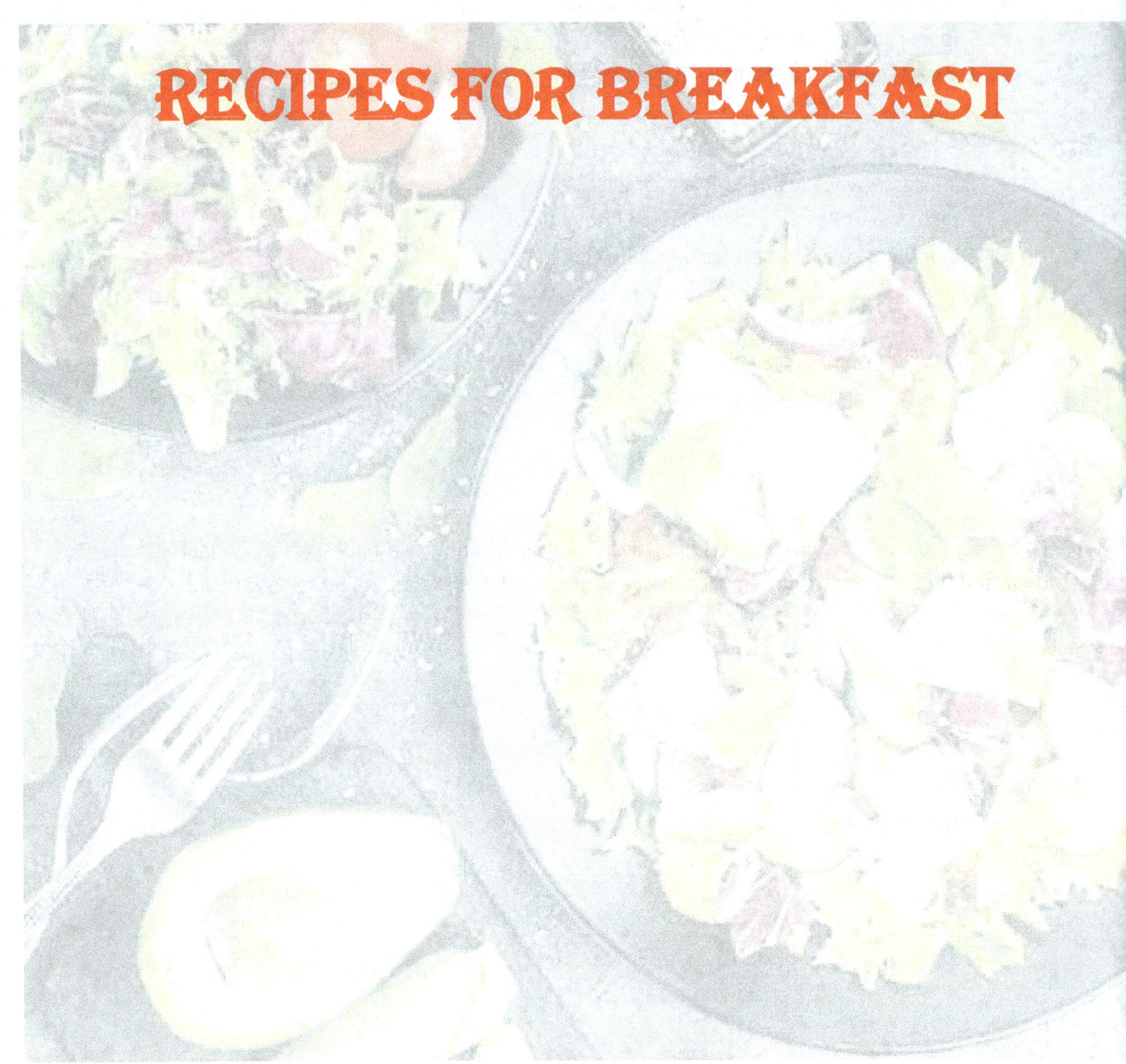

MTHFR-Friendly Smoothie Bowl

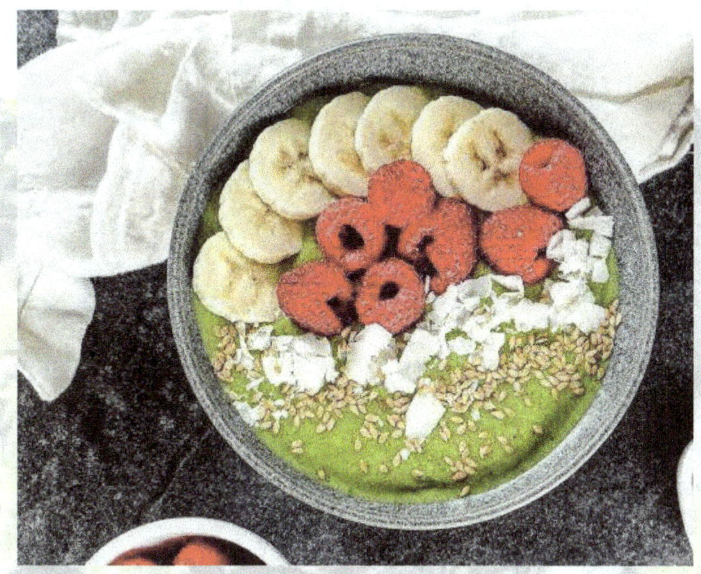

Ingredients:

- 1 cup organic spinach leaves
- 1/2 cup blueberries (fresh or frozen)
- 1/2 avocado, peeled and diced
- 1/2 cup pineapple chunks
- 1 tablespoon chia seeds
- 1 tablespoon ground flaxseed
- 1/2 cup coconut water
- 1/2 cup almond milk (unsweetened)
- 1 teaspoon spirulina powder (optional)
- 1 scoop MTHFR-friendly protein powder (look for methylated forms)

Procedure:

- Combine spinach, blueberries, avocado, pineapple, chia seeds, flaxseed, coconut water, almond milk, spirulina powder (if using), and protein powder in a blender.
- Blend until smooth and creamy.
- Pour into a bowl and garnish with your favorite toppings like sliced strawberries, coconut flakes, and additional chia seeds.

- Approximately 10 minutes.

Tips and Tricks:

- Use frozen fruits for a thicker consistency.
- Adjust the sweetness by adding a drizzle of honey or maple syrup if desired.
- Experiment with different toppings for added texture and flavor.

Nutritional Value per Serving:

- Calories: ~300
- Protein: ~15g
- Fiber: ~10g
- Healthy Fats: ~15g

- Vitamins and Minerals:

- Rich in vitamins A, C, K, and folate.

Health Benefits:

- Supports methylation processes with MTHFR-friendly nutrients.
- Provides a nutrient-dense, anti-inflammatory boost.
- Supports energy levels and overall well-being.

Packaging and Storing:

- Consume immediately for optimal freshness.
- If storing, refrigerate in an airtight container for up to 24 hours.

Estimated Cost of Preparation:

- Varies based on ingredient quality and location. Typically ranges from $10 to $15 per serving.

Precautions:

- Consult a healthcare professional before introducing new supplements or ingredients, especially for those with MTHFR variations.
- Be mindful of potential allergies to any of the ingredients.

- Listen to your body and adjust ingredients as needed.
- Regularly review and update the recipe based on personal health goals and dietary requirements.

Quinoa and Vegetable Breakfast Bowl

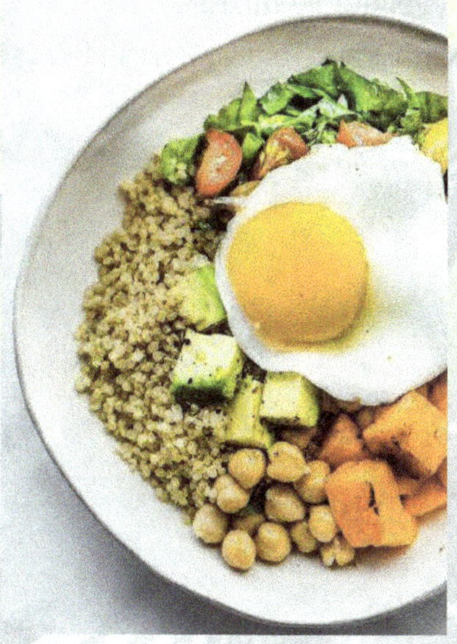

Ingredients:

- 1 cup quinoa, rinsed
- 2 cups water or vegetable broth
- 1 tablespoon olive oil
- 1 onion, diced
- 2 bell peppers, diced (mix of colors)
- 1 zucchini, diced
- 1 cup cherry tomatoes, halved
- 2 cloves garlic, minced
- 1 teaspoon cumin
- Salt and pepper to taste
- 4 large eggs (optional, for topping)
- Fresh herbs (e.g., parsley or cilantro) for garnish

- In a saucepan, combine quinoa and water or vegetable broth. Bring to a boil, then reduce heat, cover, and simmer for 15-20 minutes or until quinoa is cooked and water is absorbed.
- In a large skillet, heat olive oil over medium heat. Add diced onion and cook until translucent.
- Add bell peppers, zucchini, cherry tomatoes, minced garlic, cumin, salt, and pepper to the skillet. Cook until vegetables are tender yet still vibrant.
- Stir in cooked quinoa, ensuring all ingredients are well combined. Cook for an additional 2-3 minutes to allow flavors to meld.
- If desired, fry eggs in a separate pan to top the quinoa and vegetable mixture.
- Serve the quinoa and vegetable mixture in bowls, topping with a fried egg and fresh herbs.

Time of Preparation:

- Approximately 30 minutes.

Tips and Tricks:

- Cook quinoa in vegetable broth for added flavor.
- Customize with your favorite vegetables or add avocado for extra creaminess.
- Experiment with different spices to suit your taste preferences.

Nutritional Value per Serving:

- Calories: ~400
- Protein: ~15g
- Fiber: ~8g
- Healthy Fats: ~10g
- Rich in vitamins A, C, and K, as well as iron and magnesium.

Health Benefits:

- High protein and fiber content for sustained energy.
- Packed with essential vitamins and minerals for overall well-being.
- Provides a balanced and nutritious start to the day.

Packaging and Storing:

- Store any leftovers in an airtight container in the refrigerator for up to 2 days.
- Reheat in the microwave or on the stovetop before serving.

- Varies based on ingredient quality and location. Typically ranges from $8 to $12 per serving.

- Adjust seasoning based on personal preferences and dietary restrictions.
- If using eggs, ensure they are cooked to your desired level of doneness.

- Monitor portion sizes to meet individual nutritional needs.
- Modify ingredients to suit taste preferences and dietary goals.

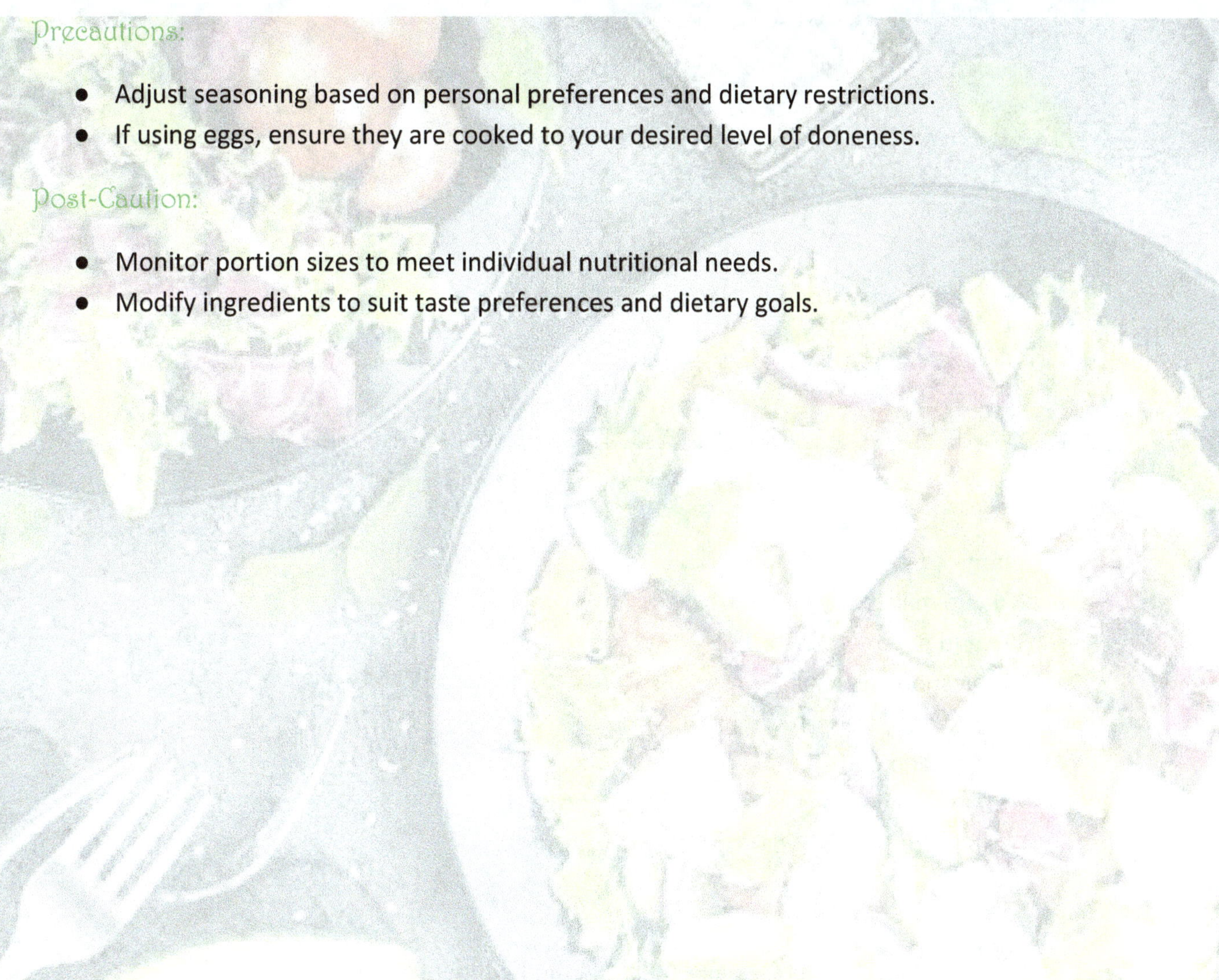

Avocado and Spinach Omelet

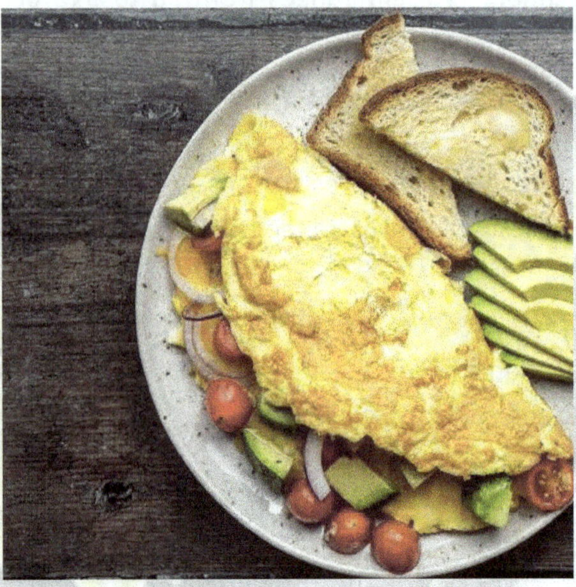

Ingredients:

- 2 large eggs
- 1/4 cup milk (dairy or plant-based)
- Salt and pepper to taste
- 1 tablespoon olive oil
- 1/2 cup baby spinach, chopped
- 1/2 avocado, sliced
- 2 tablespoons feta cheese, crumbled (optional)
- Fresh herbs (e.g., chives or parsley) for garnish

Procedure:

- In a bowl, whisk together eggs, milk, salt, and pepper until well combined.
- Heat olive oil in a non-stick skillet over medium heat.
- Add chopped baby spinach to the skillet and sauté until wilted.
- Pour the egg mixture over the spinach, ensuring an even distribution.
- Allow the eggs to set slightly at the edges, then gently lift and tilt the skillet to let the uncooked eggs flow to the edges.
- Once the omelet is mostly set but still slightly runny on top, add sliced avocado and crumbled feta (if using) to one half of the omelet.
- Carefully fold the other half over the filling, creating a half-moon shape.
- Cook for an additional 1-2 minutes until the omelet is cooked through but still moist.
- Slide the omelet onto a plate, garnish with fresh herbs, and serve immediately.

- Approximately 15 minutes.

- Use a non-stick skillet for easy flipping.
- Customize with additional veggies or protein like tomatoes, mushrooms, or cooked chicken.
- For a creamier texture, add a dollop of Greek yogurt or sour cream before folding.

- Calories: ~300
- Protein: ~15g
- Healthy Fats: ~20g
- Rich in vitamins A, C, and K, as well as potassium.

- Provides a good source of protein and healthy fats.
- Spinach offers essential vitamins and minerals.
- Avocado contributes heart-healthy monounsaturated fats.

- Best enjoyed fresh; omelets don't store well.
- If needed, store in an airtight container in the refrigerator for up to one day. Reheat gently.

- Varies based on ingredient quality and location. Typically ranges from $5 to $8 per serving.

- Adjust salt intake based on dietary preferences and health conditions.
- Be cautious when flipping the omelet to avoid breakage.

- Monitor portion sizes for balanced nutrition.
- Experiment with different fillings and toppings for variety.

CHAPTER 5

LUNCH CREATIONS

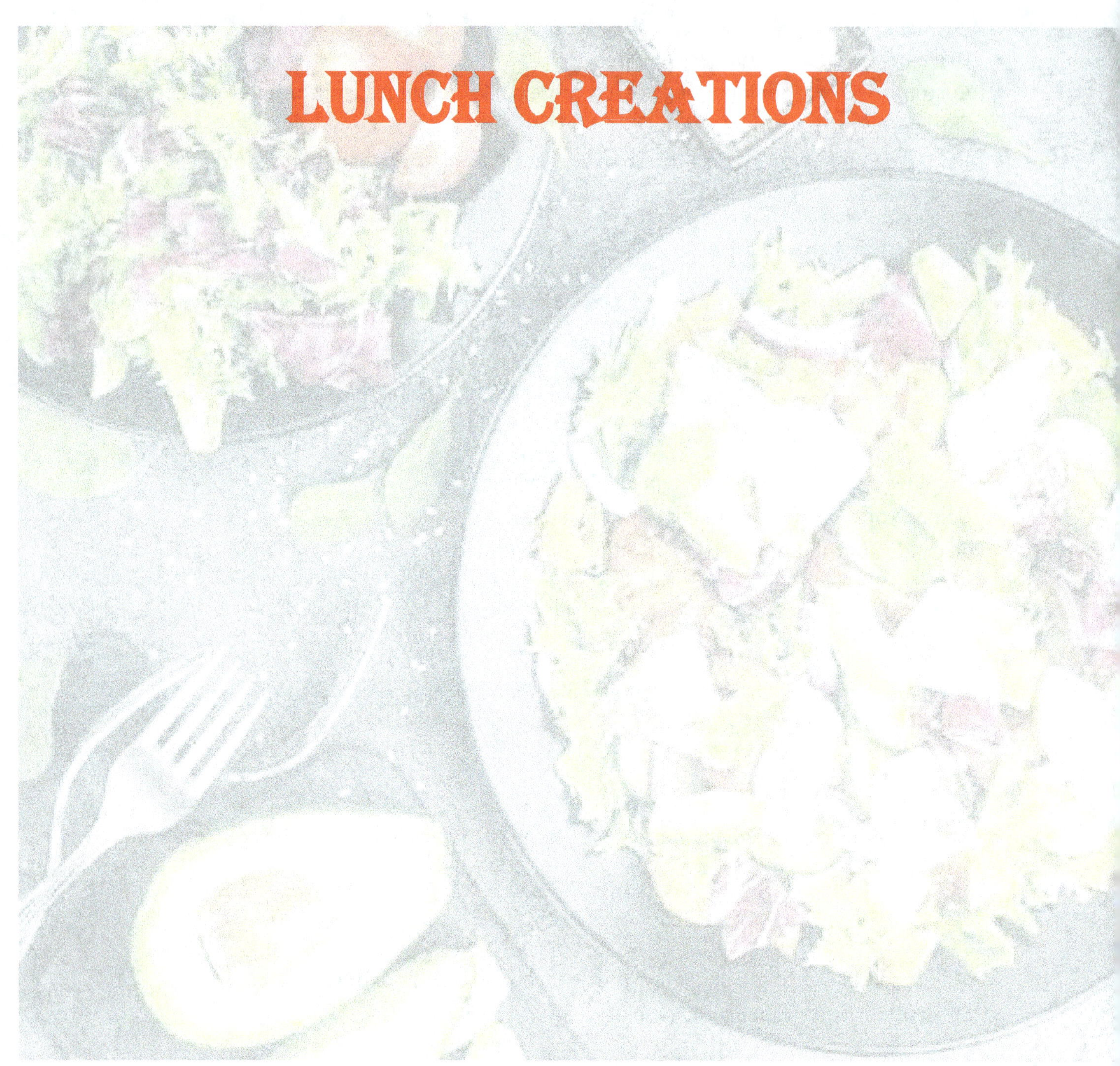

Salmon and Avocado Salad

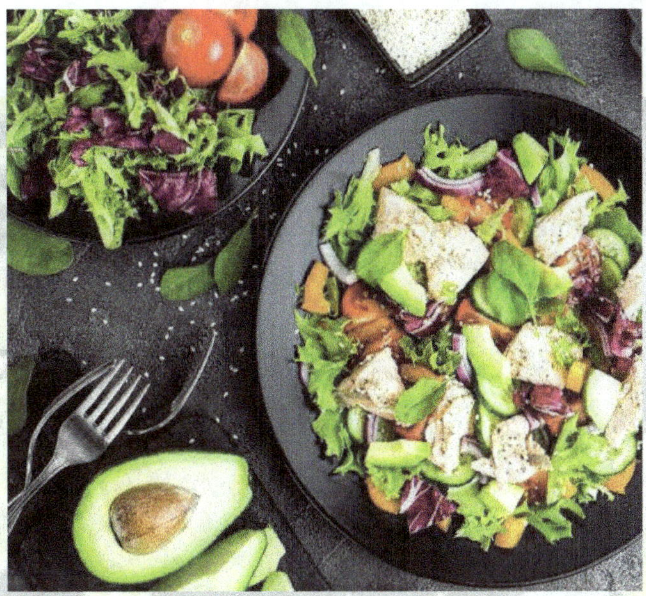

Ingredients:

- 1 pound fresh salmon filets
- 2 ripe avocados, diced
- 1 cup cherry tomatoes, halved
- 1/4 cup red onion, finely chopped
- 1/4 cup fresh cilantro, chopped
- 2 tablespoons extra-virgin olive oil
- 1 tablespoon lemon juice
- Salt and pepper to taste
- Mixed salad greens (optional)

Procedures:

- Preheat the Oven: Preheat your oven to 400°F (200°C).
- Prepare Salmon: Place salmon filets on a baking sheet lined with parchment paper. Drizzle with olive oil, lemon juice, salt, and pepper. Bake for 12-15 minutes or until salmon is cooked through and flakes easily.
- Assemble Salad: In a large bowl, combine diced avocados, cherry tomatoes, red onion, and cilantro. Gently flake the cooked salmon into the bowl.
- Dressing: Drizzle extra-virgin olive oil over the salad, add salt and pepper to taste. Toss gently to combine, ensuring the salmon and avocado are evenly coated.
- Serve: Optionally, serve the salad over a bed of mixed salad greens.

- Approximately 20-25 minutes.

- Use fresh, high-quality salmon for the best flavor.
- Adjust lemon juice and olive oil quantities to your taste preference.
- Allow the salmon to cool slightly before mixing it with the salad to prevent wilting.

Nutritional Value per Serving:

- Calories: ~350 kcal
- Protein: ~25g
- Healthy Fats: ~20g
- Carbohydrates: ~15g
- Fiber: ~7g

Health Benefits:

- Rich in Omega-3 fatty acids from salmon, promoting heart health.
- Avocado provides monounsaturated fats and various vitamins.
- High protein content supports muscle health.

Packaging and Storing:

- Store leftovers in an airtight container in the refrigerator.
- Consume within 1-2 days for optimal freshness.

Estimated Cost of Preparation:

- Depending on location and ingredient quality, approximately $15-$20.

Precautions:

- Check for any allergies among diners.
- Ensure salmon is thoroughly cooked to avoid foodborne illnesses.

Post Caution:

- Properly refrigerate any leftovers promptly.
- Reheat if necessary but avoid overcooking to maintain texture.
- Enjoy your Salmon and Avocado Salad – a nutritious and flavorful dish that's easy to prepare!

Lentil and Vegetable Wrap

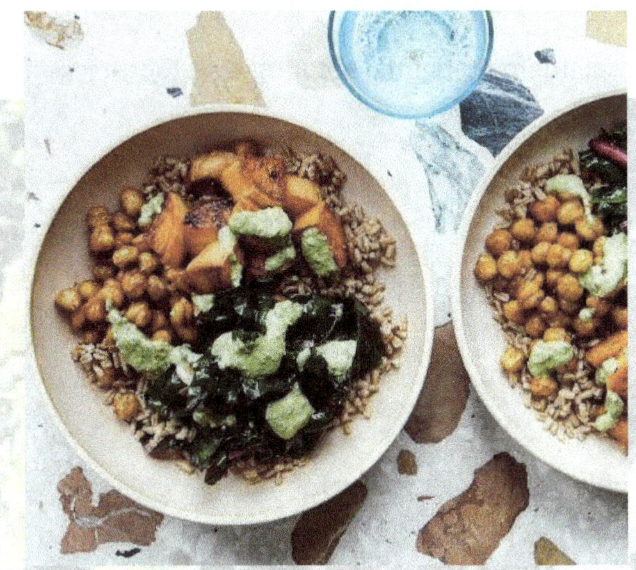

- 1 cup dry lentils, cooked
- 1 bell pepper, thinly sliced
- 1 zucchini, julienned
- 1 carrot, shredded
- 1/2 red onion, thinly sliced
- 2 cloves garlic, minced
- 2 tablespoons olive oil
- 1 teaspoon ground cumin
- 1 teaspoon paprika
- Salt and pepper to taste
- Whole wheat wraps
- Hummus for spreading
- Fresh cilantro for garnish

Procedures:

- Cook Lentils: Cook the lentils according to package instructions. Drain any excess water.
- Sauté Vegetables: In a large skillet, heat olive oil over medium heat. Sauté garlic until fragrant, then add bell pepper, zucchini, carrot, and red onion. Cook until vegetables are tender but still crisp.
- Season: Sprinkle cumin, paprika, salt, and pepper over the vegetables. Stir in the cooked lentils, ensuring they are well-coated with the seasoning.

- Prepare Wraps: Warm the whole wheat wraps. Spread a layer of hummus on each wrap.
- Assemble: Spoon the lentil and vegetable mixture onto the wraps. Garnish with fresh cilantro.
- Wrap: Fold in the sides of the wraps and roll them up tightly, securing with toothpicks if needed.

Time of Preparation:

- Approximately 30 minutes.

Tips and Tricks:

- Experiment with different hummus flavors for added variety.
- Use whole wheat wraps for a healthier option.
- Customize with your favorite veggies or add a squeeze of lemon for freshness.

Nutritional Value per Serving:

- Calories: ~400 kcal
- Protein: ~18g
- Fiber: ~10g
- Healthy Fats: ~12g
- Carbohydrates: ~60g

Health Benefits:

- High fiber content promotes digestive health.
- Lentils are a good source of plant-based protein.
- Abundance of vitamins and minerals from vegetables.

Packaging and Storing:

- Wrap tightly in parchment or foil for easy handling.
- Ideal for meal prepping; store wrapped lentil and vegetable wraps in the refrigerator.

Estimated Cost of Preparation:

- Budget-friendly at approximately $10-$15, depending on ingredient prices.

Precautions:

- Be cautious with toothpicks when securing wraps to avoid accidents.
- Check for any allergies among diners.

- Store leftover wraps promptly in the refrigerator.
- Reheat gently to preserve the wrap's texture.
- Enjoy your Lentil and Vegetable Wrap – a wholesome and satisfying meal filled with nutritious goodness!

Sweet Potato and Chickpea Buddha Bowl

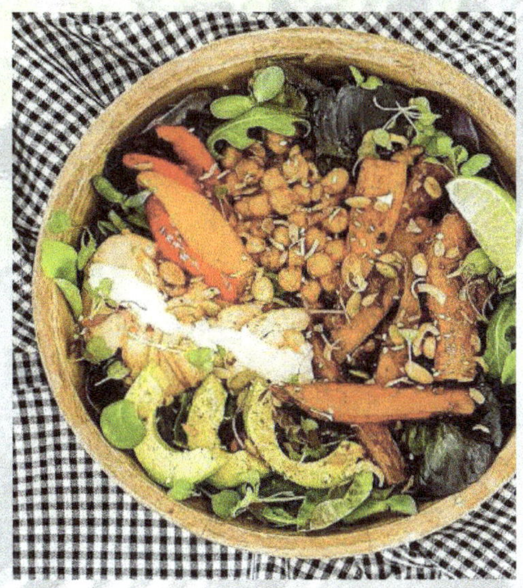

Ingredients:

- 2 medium sweet potatoes, cubed
- 1 can (15 oz) chickpeas, drained and rinsed
- 1 tablespoon olive oil
- 1 teaspoon smoked paprika
- 1 teaspoon cumin
- Salt and pepper to taste
- 2 cups quinoa, cooked
- 2 cups kale, chopped
- 1 avocado, sliced
- 1/4 cup tahini
- Lemon wedges for serving

- Roast Sweet Potatoes and Chickpeas:
- Preheat the oven to 425°F (220°C). Toss sweet potato cubes and chickpeas with olive oil, smoked paprika, cumin, salt, and pepper. Roast for 25-30 minutes until golden and crispy.

- Prepare Quinoa: Cook quinoa according to package instructions.
- Sauté Kale: In a skillet, sauté chopped kale until wilted, about 3-5 minutes.
- Assemble Buddha Bowl: Divide cooked quinoa among bowls. Top with roasted sweet potatoes and chickpeas, sautéed kale, and sliced avocado.
- Drizzle with Tahini: Drizzle tahini over the Buddha bowls.
- Serve with Lemon Wedges: Serve with lemon wedges for an extra burst of freshness.

Time of Preparation:

- Approximately 45 minutes.

Tips and Tricks:

- Customize with your favorite veggies or add a sprinkle of nutritional yeast for extra flavor.
- Drizzle tahini just before serving to maintain its creamy texture.
- Experiment with different spices for roasted sweet potatoes and chickpeas.

Nutritional Value per Serving:

- Calories: ~500 kcal
- Protein: ~15g
- Fiber: ~12g
- Healthy Fats: ~20g
- Carbohydrates: ~70g

Health Benefits:

- Sweet potatoes provide beta-carotene and fiber.
- Chickpeas are a good source of plant-based protein.
- Kale adds vitamins A, K, and C to the dish.

Packaging and Storing:

- Store components separately to maintain freshness.
- Assemble Buddha bowl just before serving.

- Cost-effective at around $12-$15, depending on ingredient prices.

- Be cautious with hot oven trays and pans.
- Check for any allergies among diners.

- Store leftover components separately in airtight containers.
- Reheat chickpeas and sweet potatoes in the oven for crispiness.
- Enjoy your Sweet Potato and Chickpea Buddha Bowl – a nutrient-packed and delicious meal for a balanced and wholesome dining experience!

CHAPTER 6

NOURISHING SNACKS

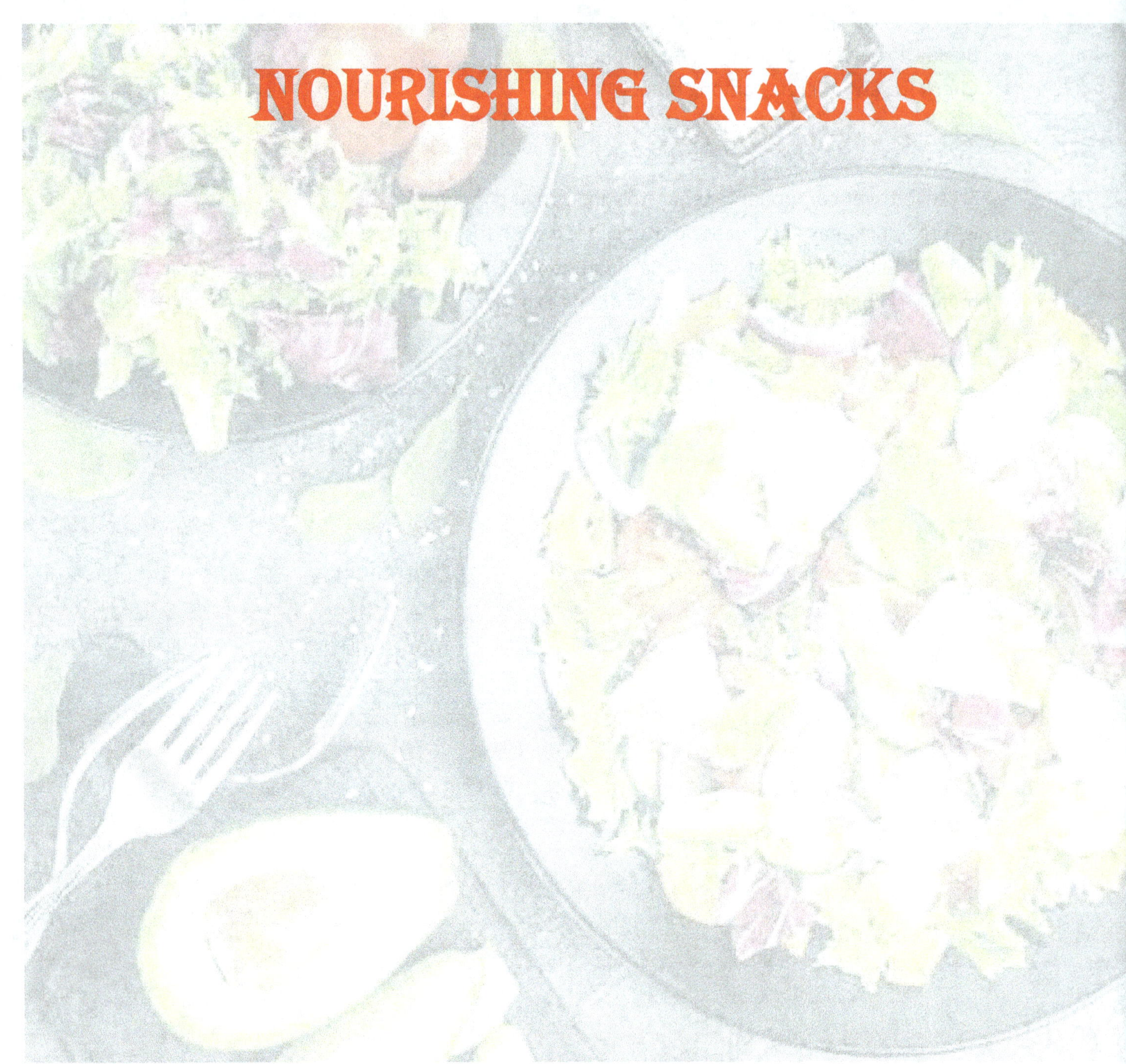

Almond and Chia Seed Energy Bites

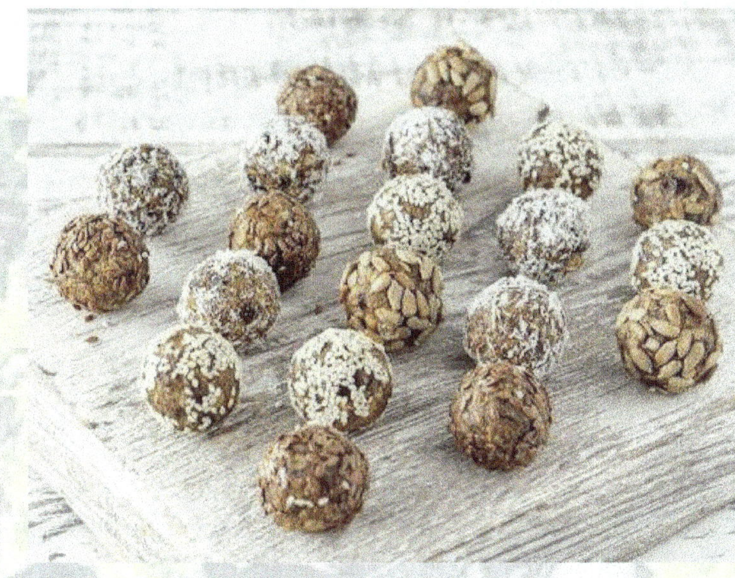

Ingredients:

- 1 cup almonds (raw or lightly roasted)
- 1/2 cup chia seeds
- 1/2 cup rolled oats
- 1/4 cup honey or maple syrup
- 1/4 cup almond butter
- 1 teaspoon vanilla extract
- A pinch of salt

- Optional: dark chocolate chips or dried fruits for added sweetness

Procedure:

- In a food processor, combine almonds, chia seeds, and rolled oats. Pulse until finely ground.
- Add honey or maple syrup, almond butter, vanilla extract, and a pinch of salt. Blend until the mixture forms a sticky dough.
- If desired, fold in dark chocolate chips or dried fruits for extra flavor and texture.
- Using your hands, roll the mixture into bite-sized balls and place them on a parchment-lined tray.
- Chill in the refrigerator for at least 30 minutes to firm up.

- Approximately 15 minutes (excluding chilling time).

Tips and Tricks:

- Roasting almonds before blending can enhance the flavor.
- Adjust sweetness by varying the amount of honey or adding more chocolate chips.
- Wet your hands slightly to prevent the mixture from sticking when rolling.

Nutritional Value per Serving:

- Calories: ~150
- Protein: 4g
- Fiber: 3g
- Healthy fats: 10g
- Carbohydrates: 12g

Health Benefits:

- Rich in omega-3 fatty acids from chia seeds for heart health.
- Almonds provide a good source of protein and vitamin E.
- Chia seeds contribute fiber and help in hydration.

Packaging and Storing:

- Store in an airtight container in the refrigerator for up to two weeks.
- For longer shelf life, freeze the energy bites and thaw before consuming.

Estimated Cost of Preparation:

- $10 - $15 for a batch of 20 bites.

Precautions:

- Be cautious if allergic to nuts or seeds.
- Check the consistency of the mixture; add more oats if too sticky or more honey if too dry.

Post-Caution:

- Enjoy these energy bites as a healthy snack but consume in moderation due to the calorie content.
- Share and store responsibly to maintain freshness.

- These Almond and Chia Seed Energy Bites are a nutritious and convenient snack, providing a balance of protein, healthy fats, and fiber for sustained energy throughout the day.

Greek Yogurt Parfait with Berries

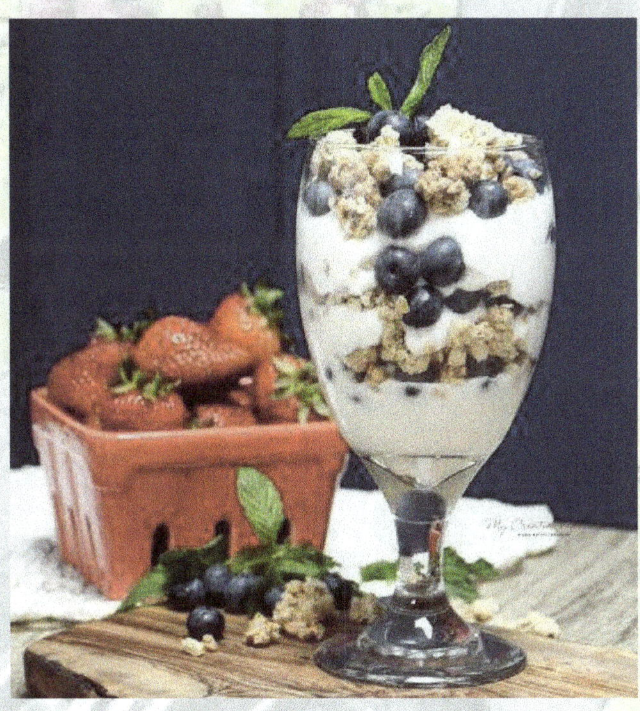

Ingredients:

- 1 cup Greek yogurt (plain or flavored)
- 1/2 cup granola
- 1/2 cup mixed berries (strawberries, blueberries, raspberries)
- 1 tablespoon honey or maple syrup
- 1/4 cup nuts (almonds, walnuts) for crunch (optional)
- Fresh mint leaves for garnish (optional)

Procedure:

- In a glass or bowl, layer the bottom with Greek yogurt.
- Add a layer of granola, followed by a layer of mixed berries.
- Drizzle honey or maple syrup over the berries.

- Repeat the layers until the glass or bowl is filled.
- Top with nuts for added crunch and garnish with fresh mint leaves.

Time of Preparation:

- Approximately 10 minutes.

Tips and Tricks:

- Use thick Greek yogurt for a creamy texture.
- Experiment with different flavored yogurts for variety.
- Toast the nuts lightly for enhanced flavor.

Nutritional Value per Serving:

- Calories: ~300
- Protein: 15g
- Fiber: 5g
- Calcium: 20% of daily value
- Antioxidants from berries for immune support.

Health Benefits:

- Greek yogurt provides probiotics for gut health.
- Berries are rich in vitamins, antioxidants, and fiber.
- Nuts offer healthy fats and additional protein.

Packaging and Storing:

- Serve immediately for the best texture.
- If preparing in advance, store ingredients separately and assemble just before serving.
- Refrigerate any leftovers; consume within 24 hours for optimal freshness.

Estimated Cost of Preparation:

- $5 - $8 per serving.

Precautions:

- Check yogurt expiration date for freshness.
- Be cautious with portion sizes, as the granola and flavored yogurt can contribute to calorie intake.

- Enjoy this Greek Yogurt Parfait as a wholesome breakfast or snack.
- Customize with different fruits, nuts, or seeds based on dietary preferences.
- Watch portion sizes if incorporating into a calorie-controlled diet.

Nut and Seed Trail Mix

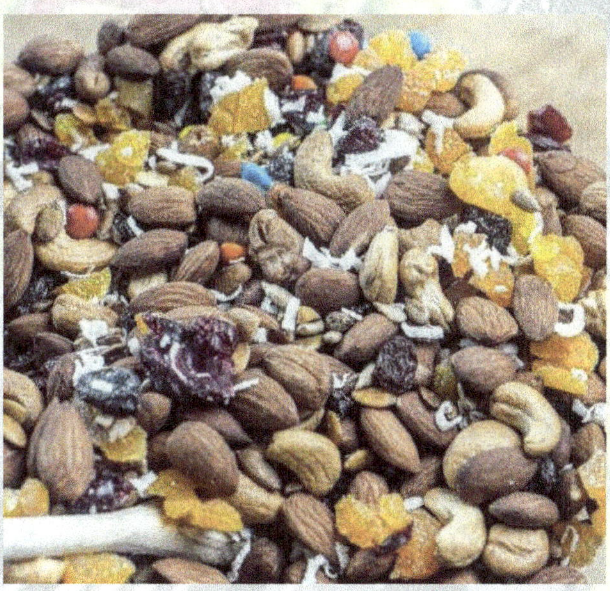

Ingredients:

- 1 cup almonds
- 1/2 cup walnuts
- 1/2 cup pumpkin seeds
- 1/4 cup sunflower seeds
- 1/4 cup cashews
- 1/4 cup dried cranberries
- 1/4 cup dark chocolate chips
- 1 teaspoon cinnamon
- A pinch of salt

- In a dry skillet over medium heat, lightly toast almonds, walnuts, pumpkin seeds, sunflower seeds, and cashews until fragrant. Allow them to cool.
- In a mixing bowl, combine the toasted nuts and seeds with dried cranberries, dark chocolate chips, cinnamon, and a pinch of salt.
- Toss the mixture until well combined.
- Allow the trail mix to cool completely before storing in an airtight container.

Time of Preparation:

- Approximately 15 minutes (excluding cooling time).

Tips and Tricks:

- Customize the mix with your favorite nuts, seeds, or dried fruits.
- Adjust sweetness by varying the amount of chocolate chips.
- Store in single-serving bags for convenient, on-the-go snacks.

Nutritional Value per Serving:

- Calories: ~200
- Protein: 7g
- Healthy fats: 15g
- Fiber: 3g
- Rich in antioxidants, vitamins, and minerals.

Health Benefits:

- Nuts and seeds provide heart-healthy fats and essential nutrients.
- Dark chocolate contributes antioxidants and may improve mood.
- Pumpkin seeds are a good source of magnesium for muscle and nerve function.

Packaging and Storing:

- Store in an airtight container in a cool, dry place.
- Portion into small bags for a convenient grab-and-go snack.
- Keep away from direct sunlight to maintain freshness.

Estimated Cost of Preparation:

- $10 - $12 for a batch.

- Be cautious if allergic to nuts or seeds.
- Monitor portion sizes to avoid excessive calorie intake.

- Enjoy this Nut and Seed Trail Mix as a nutritious snack.
- Incorporate into your diet for a quick energy boost.
- Share with caution, especially if allergies are a concern among friends or family.

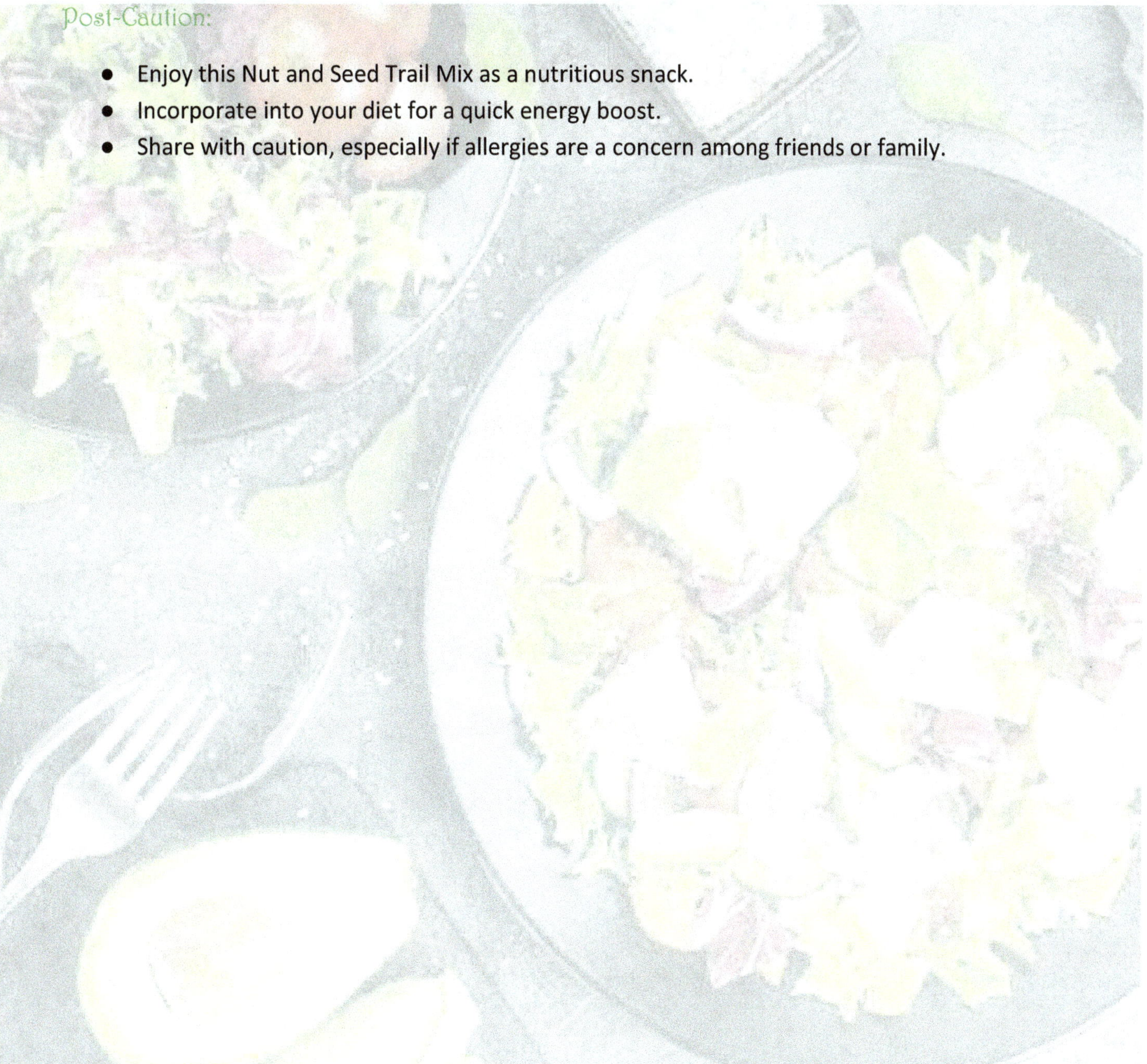

CHAPTER 7

DINNER DELIGHTS

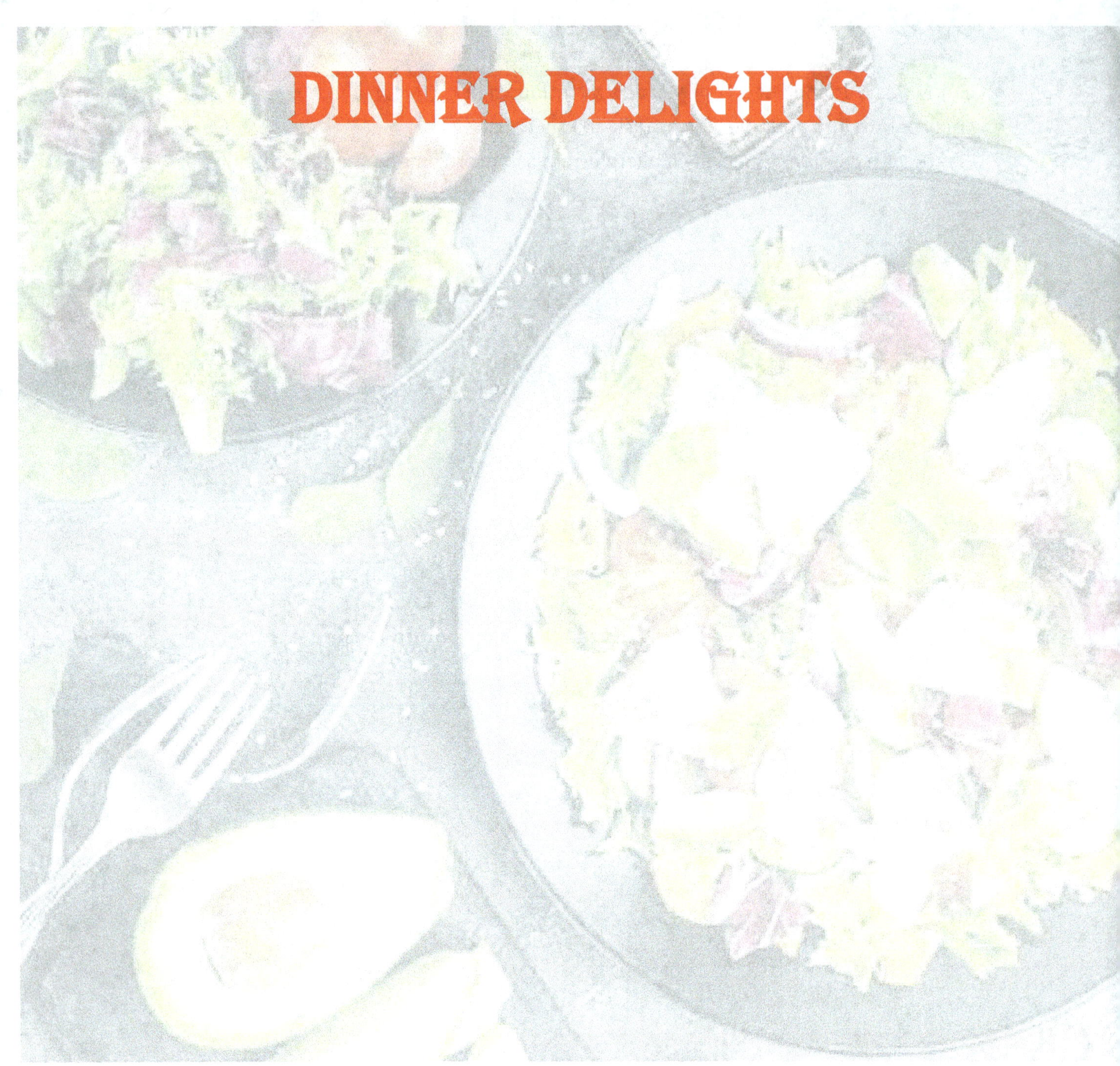

Baked Salmon with Lemon and Dill

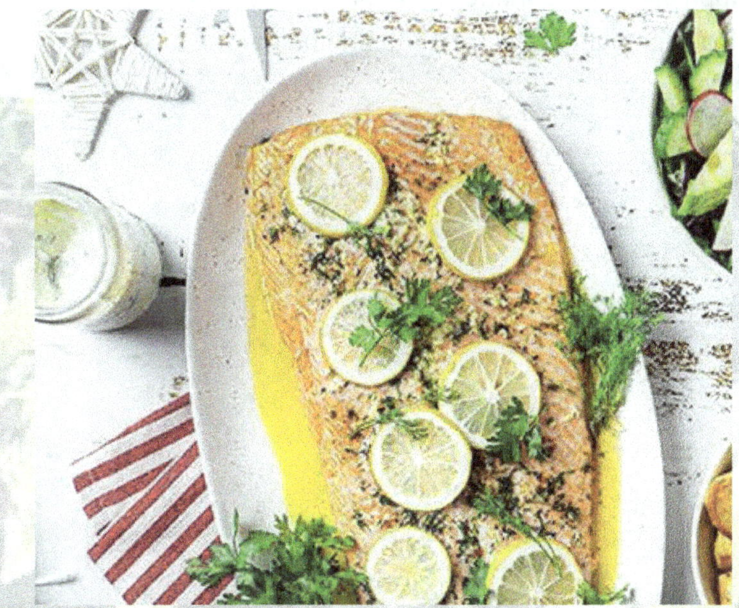

Ingredients:

- 4 salmon filets
- 1/4 cup olive oil
- 2 tablespoons fresh lemon juice
- 2 cloves garlic, minced
- 1 tablespoon fresh dill, chopped
- Salt and pepper to taste
- Lemon slices for garnish

Procedure:

- Preheat the oven to 375°F (190°C).
- Place the salmon filets on a baking sheet lined with parchment paper.
- In a small bowl, mix olive oil, lemon juice, minced garlic, chopped dill, salt, and pepper to create the marinade.
- Brush the marinade over the salmon filets, ensuring even coverage.
- Place lemon slices on top of each filet for added flavor.
- Bake in the preheated oven for 15-20 minutes or until the salmon easily flakes with a fork.
- Garnish with additional fresh dill before serving.

Time of Preparation:

- Approximately 30 minutes

- Pat the salmon filets dry before applying the marinade to enhance the flavors.
- For extra moisture, cover the baking sheet with foil during the first half of the baking time.

Nutritional Value per Serving:

- Calories: 300
- Protein: 25g
- Fat: 20g
- Carbohydrates: 2g
- Fiber: 1g

Health Benefits:

- Rich in omega-3 fatty acids for heart health.
- High in protein for muscle development.
- Dill provides antioxidants and has anti-inflammatory properties.

Packaging and Storing:

- Store leftovers in an airtight container in the refrigerator for up to 2 days.
- To freeze, wrap individual filets in plastic wrap and place in a freezer bag for up to 2 months.

Estimated Cost of Preparation:

- $15-$20 (may vary based on location and ingredient quality)

Precautions:

- Ensure the salmon reaches an internal temperature of 145°F (63°C) to guarantee its safety for consumption.
- Be cautious with cross-contamination; clean utensils and surfaces after handling raw fish.

Post Caution:

- Discard any leftovers that have been left at room temperature for more than 2 hours to prevent foodborne illnesses.
- Be mindful of potential allergies to fish and adjust the recipe accordingly.

Quinoa-Stuffed Bell Peppers

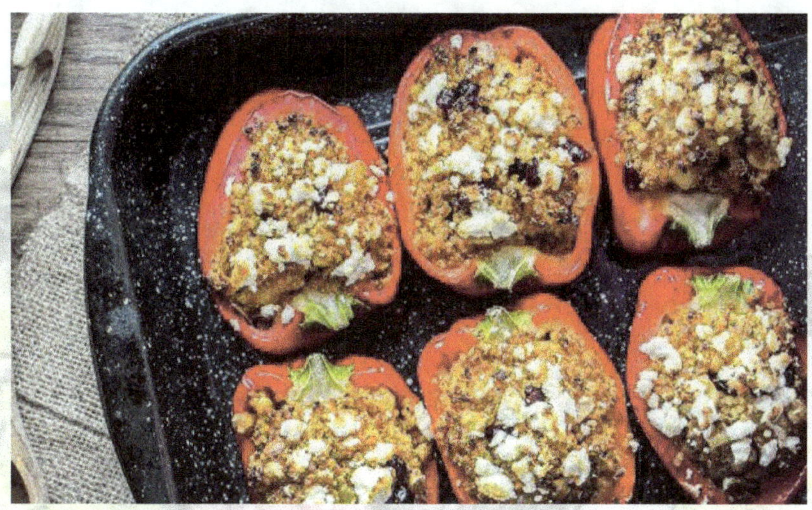

Ingredients:

- 4 large bell peppers (any color)
- 1 cup quinoa, rinsed
- 2 cups vegetable broth
- 1 can (15 oz) black beans, drained and rinsed
- 1 cup corn kernels (fresh or frozen)
- 1 cup cherry tomatoes, diced
- 1/2 cup red onion, finely chopped
- 1 teaspoon ground cumin
- 1 teaspoon chili powder
- 1/2 teaspoon garlic powder
- Salt and pepper to taste
- 1 cup shredded cheese (optional, for topping)
- Fresh cilantro or parsley for garnish

Procedure:

- Preheat the oven to 375°F (190°C).
- Cut the tops off the bell peppers, remove seeds and membranes.
- In a saucepan, combine quinoa and vegetable broth. Bring to a boil, then reduce heat and simmer for 15-20 minutes until quinoa is cooked and water is absorbed.
- In a large bowl, mix cooked quinoa, black beans, corn, cherry tomatoes, red onion, cumin, chili powder, garlic powder, salt, and pepper.
- Stuff each bell pepper with the quinoa mixture.
- Place stuffed peppers in a baking dish, cover with foil, and bake for 25-30 minutes.

- If desired, top each pepper with shredded cheese and bake for an additional 5 minutes until melted.
- Garnish with fresh cilantro or parsley before serving.

Time of Preparation:

- Approximately 45 minutes

Tips and Tricks:

- Partially cook the bell peppers in boiling water for 5 minutes before stuffing to reduce baking time.
- Customize the filing with your favorite vegetables or add protein like cooked ground turkey or chicken.

Nutritional Value per Serving:

- Calories: 350
- Protein: 12g
- Fat: 6g
- Carbohydrates: 65g
- Fiber: 12g

Health Benefits:

- Quinoa provides complete protein and is rich in fiber.
- Bell peppers are high in vitamin C and antioxidants.
- Black beans offer a good source of protein and fiber.

Packaging and Storing:

- Store leftovers in an airtight container in the refrigerator for up to 3 days.
- Reheat in the oven or microwave for a quick and healthy meal.

Estimated Cost of Preparation:

- $12-$15 (may vary based on location and ingredient quality)

Precautions:

- Ensure bell peppers are thoroughly cooked to a soft texture.
- Check for any allergies to quinoa or other ingredients.

- Discard any leftovers that have been left at room temperature for more than 2 hours to avoid bacterial growth.
- Be cautious with reheating to maintain optimal taste and texture.

Turmeric Chicken Stir-fry

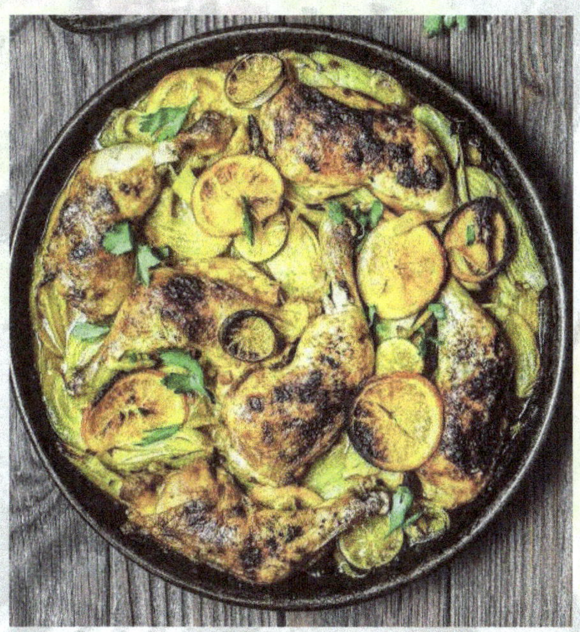

Ingredients:

- 1 lb boneless, skinless chicken breasts, thinly sliced
- 2 tablespoons soy sauce
- 1 tablespoon turmeric powder
- 1 tablespoon honey
- 2 tablespoons sesame oil
- 1 tablespoon ginger, minced
- 2 cloves garlic, minced
- 1 red bell pepper, thinly sliced
- 1 cup broccoli florets
- 1 carrot, julienned
- 2 cups cooked brown rice or quinoa

- Green onions and sesame seeds for garnish

Procedure:

- In a bowl, combine sliced chicken with soy sauce, turmeric powder, and honey. Let it marinate for at least 15 minutes.
- Heat sesame oil in a large pan or wok over medium-high heat.
- Add ginger and garlic, stir-frying for about 30 seconds until fragrant.
- Add marinated chicken to the pan, stir-fry until fully cooked and golden brown.
- Add bell pepper, broccoli, and carrot to the pan, stir-fry for an additional 3-5 minutes until vegetables are tender-crisp.
- Serve the stir-fry over cooked brown rice or quinoa.
- Garnish with green onions and sesame seeds before serving.

Time of Preparation:

- Approximately 30 minutes

Tips and Tricks:

- Ensure the chicken is thinly sliced for quicker cooking and more even flavor distribution.
- Use a preheated wok or pan to achieve a good sear on the chicken.

Nutritional Value per Serving:

- Calories: 400
- Protein: 25g
- Fat: 10g
- Carbohydrates: 50g
- Fiber: 6g

Health Benefits:

- Turmeric has anti-inflammatory properties and adds a warm, earthy flavor.
- Chicken is a lean source of protein.
- Colorful vegetables contribute essential vitamins and minerals.

Packaging and Storing:

- Store leftovers in an airtight container in the refrigerator for up to 3 days.
- Reheat in a pan or microwave for a quick and nutritious meal.

- $15-$20 (may vary based on location and ingredient quality)

Precautions:

- Ensure the chicken reaches an internal temperature of 165°F (74°C) for safe consumption.
- Be cautious with turmeric stains on clothing and kitchen surfaces.

Post Caution:

- Discard any leftovers that have been left at room temperature for more than 2 hours to prevent bacterial growth.
- Store leftover stir-fry away from strong odors in the refrigerator to maintain freshness.

CHAPTER 8

SATISFYING SIDES

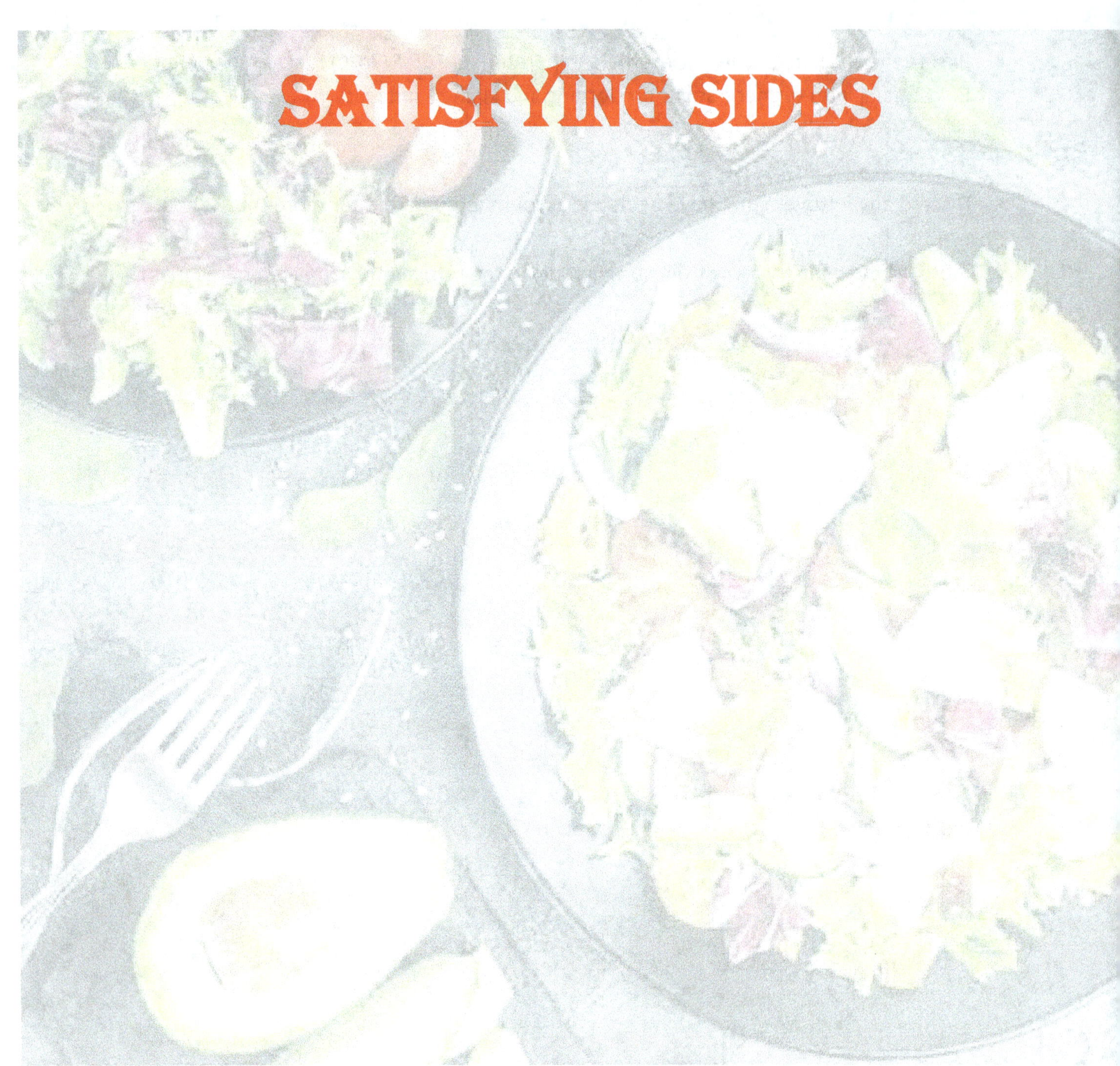

Roasted Brussels Sprouts with Garlic

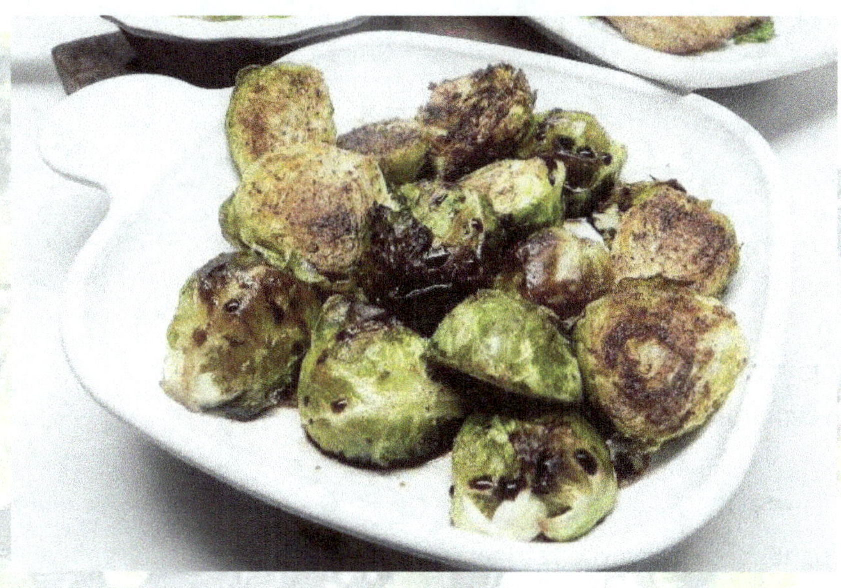

Ingredients:

- 1 lb Brussels sprouts, trimmed and halved
- 3 cloves garlic, minced
- 2 tablespoons olive oil
- Salt and pepper to taste

Procedure:

- Preheat the oven to 400°F (200°C).
- In a large bowl, toss Brussels sprouts and minced garlic with olive oil until evenly coated.
- Spread the Brussels sprouts in a single layer on a baking sheet.
- Season with salt and pepper according to your taste.
- Roast in the preheated oven for 20-25 minutes or until the sprouts are golden brown and crispy on the edges.

Time of Preparation:

- Approximately 30 minutes.

Tips and Tricks:

- Ensure the Brussels sprouts are dry before roasting for better crispiness.
- Toss halfway through roasting for even cooking.

- Add a squeeze of lemon juice for a citrusy twist.

Nutritional Value (per serving):

- Calories: 120
- Protein: 5g
- Fiber: 5g
- Vitamin C: 120% DV
- Iron: 10% DV

Health Benefits:

- High in fiber and vitamins, promoting digestive health.
- Rich in antioxidants, supporting immune function.
- Low in calories, aiding weight management.

Packaging and Storing:

- Store leftovers in an airtight container in the refrigerator for up to 3 days.
- Reheat in the oven or toaster oven for best results.

Estimated Cost of Preparation:

- $8-$10

Precautions:

- Be cautious when handling hot baking sheets.
- Ensure the Brussels sprouts are trimmed properly to avoid bitter flavors.

Post Caution:

- Consume in moderation to avoid overconsumption of fats.
- Adapt portion sizes based on individual dietary needs.

Cauliflower Mash

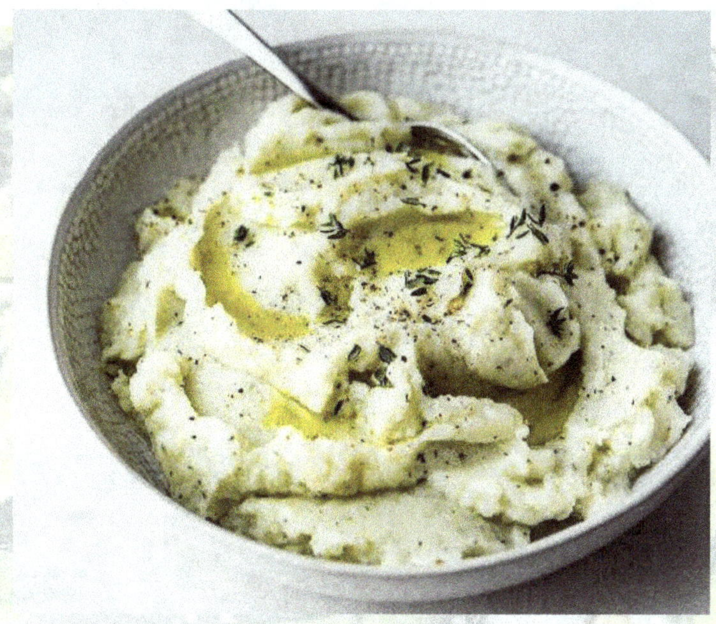

Ingredients:

- 1 head cauliflower, cut into florets
- 2 cloves garlic, minced
- 2 tablespoons butter
- 1/4 cup milk (or vegetable broth for a dairy-free option)
- Salt and pepper to taste

Procedure:

- Steam or boil cauliflower florets until tender.
- In a food processor, combine cooked cauliflower, minced garlic, butter, and milk.
- Blend until smooth and creamy.
- Season with salt and pepper according to your taste.

Time of Preparation:

- Approximately 20-25 minutes.

Tips and Tricks:

- Dry the cauliflower thoroughly after cooking to avoid a watery mash.
- Experiment with adding herbs like thyme or chives for extra flavor.

- Adjust the consistency by adding more milk or broth if needed.

Nutritional Value (per serving):

- Calories: 80
- Protein: 3g
- Fiber: 4g
- Vitamin C: 70% DV
- Potassium: 15% DV

Health Benefits:

- Low in calories and carbohydrates, suitable for low-carb diets.
- High in fiber, promoting digestive health.
- Rich in vitamin C and antioxidants, supporting immune function.

Packaging and Storing:

- Store in an airtight container in the refrigerator for up to 3 days.
- Reheat on the stovetop or in the microwave.

Estimated Cost of Preparation:

- $5-$7

Precautions:

- Be cautious when processing hot cauliflower to avoid burns.
- Check the consistency during blending to achieve the desired texture.

Post Caution:

- Be mindful of portion sizes, especially for those on low-carb diets.
- Monitor sodium intake if adding salt, considering dietary restrictions

Sauteed Kale with Pine Nuts

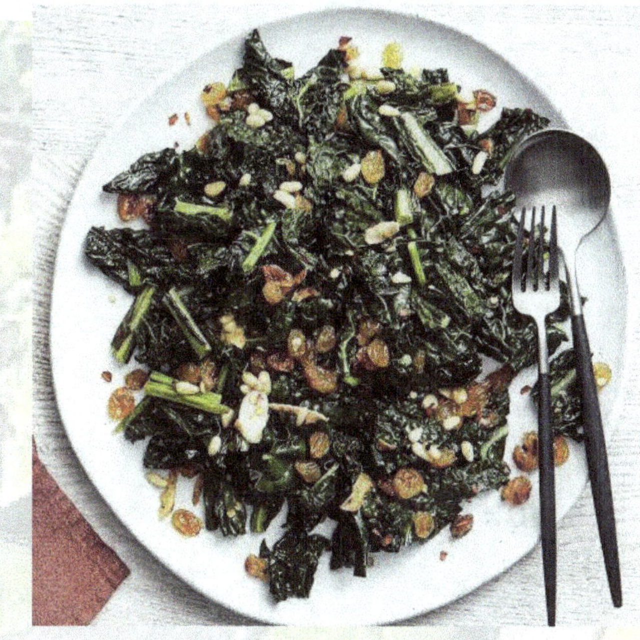

Ingredients:

- 1 bunch kale, stems removed and leaves chopped
- 2 tablespoons olive oil
- 2 cloves garlic, minced
- 1/4 cup pine nuts
- Salt and pepper to taste
- Lemon wedges for serving (optional)

Procedure:

- Heat olive oil in a large skillet over medium heat.
- Add minced garlic and sauté for 1-2 minutes until fragrant.
- Add chopped kale to the skillet and sauté until wilted but still vibrant green.
- Stir in pine nuts and continue cooking until they are lightly toasted.
- Season with salt and pepper to taste.
- Serve with a squeeze of lemon if desired.

Time of Preparation:

- Approximately 15-20 minutes.

- Massage kale leaves with olive oil before cooking to enhance tenderness.
- Toast pine nuts in a dry skillet before adding to intensify their flavor.
- Adjust seasoning based on personal preference.

Nutritional Value (per serving):

- Calories: 150
- Protein: 5g
- Fiber: 4g
- Vitamin A: 180% DV
- Vitamin C: 120% DV

Health Benefits:

- Kale is rich in vitamins A, C, and K, promoting bone and skin health.
- Pine nuts provide healthy fats and essential minerals.
- High fiber content supports digestive health.

Packaging and Storing:

- Store leftovers in an airtight container in the refrigerator for up to 2 days.
- Reheat on the stovetop or in the microwave.
- Estimated Cost of Preparation: $6-$8

Precautions:

- Exercise caution when toasting pine nuts to avoid burning.
- Monitor garlic to prevent it from becoming overly browned, which can result in bitterness.

Post Caution:

- Be mindful of portion sizes to control calorie intake.
- Check for allergies to nuts before serving to others.

CHAPTER 9

DESSERTS FOR FERTILITY

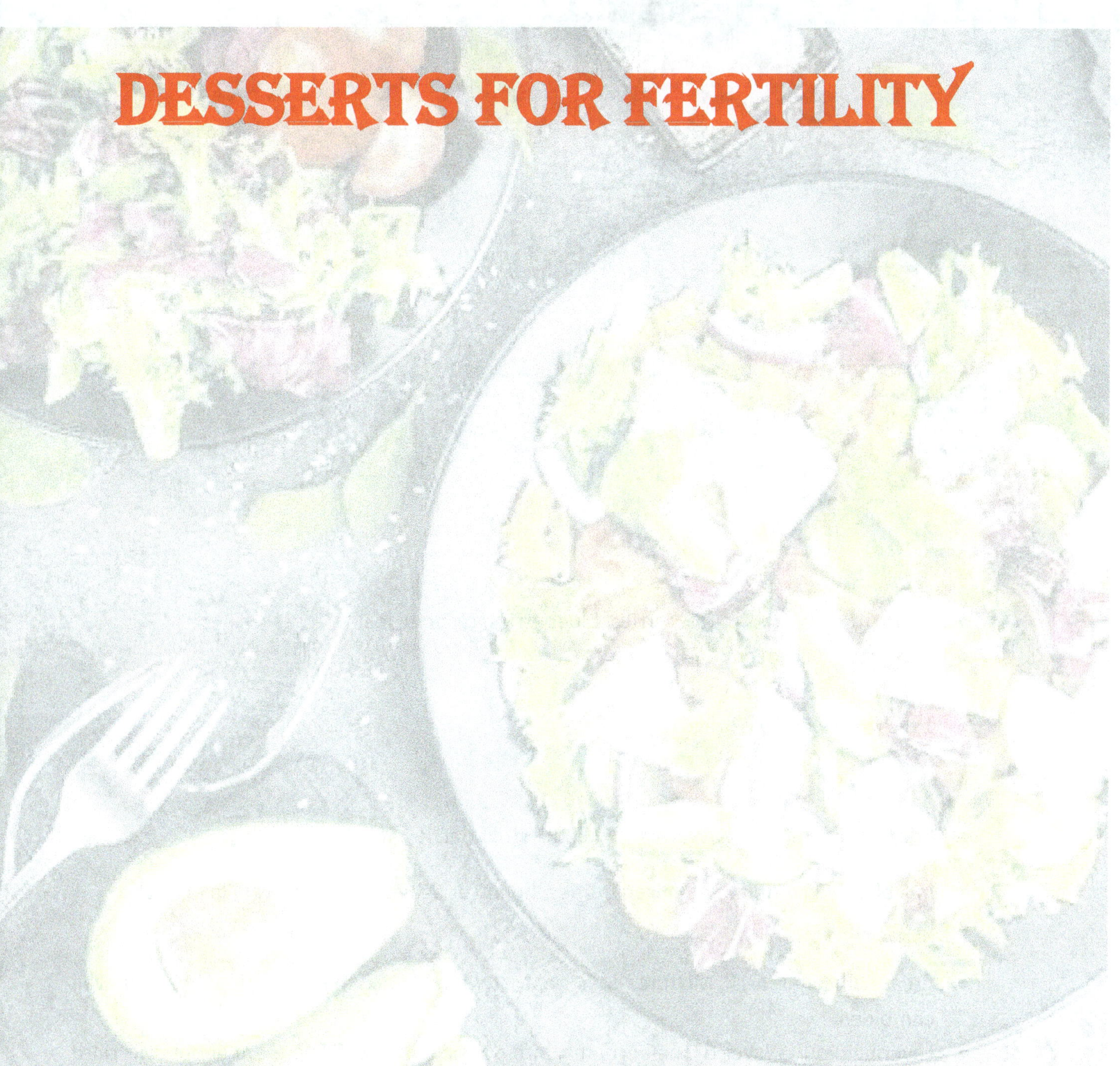

Berry and Coconut Milk Popsicles\

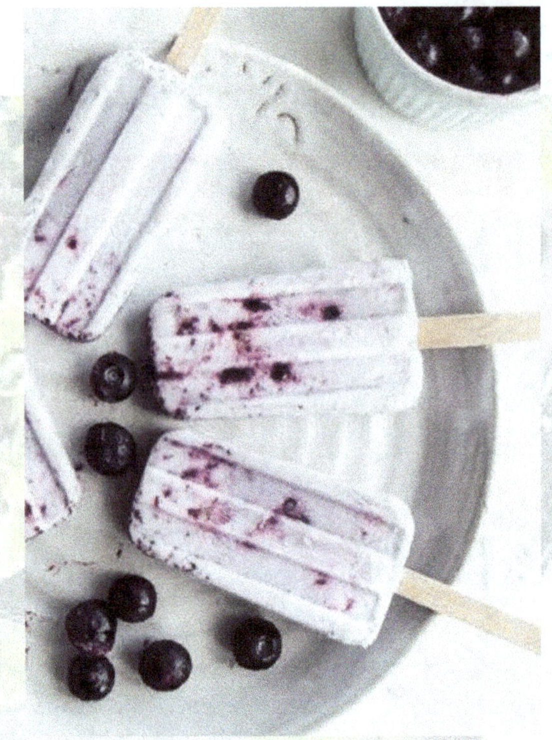

Ingredients:

- 1 cup mixed berries (strawberries, blueberries, raspberries)
- 1 can (13.5 oz) coconut milk
- 1/4 cup honey or agave syrup
- 1 teaspoon vanilla extract

Procedure:

- Prepare the Berry Mix: Wash and hull the strawberries, if using.

- In a blender, combine the mixed berries, honey or agave syrup, and vanilla extract.
- Blend until smooth.

- Create Coconut Milk Mixture: In a separate bowl, mix the coconut milk until well combined.
- Layering: Pour a layer of the berry mix into popsicle molds, filling them about one-third of the way.

- Add a layer of coconut milk on top.
- Repeat until the molds are filled.

- Freezing: Insert popsicle sticks into the molds.

- Freeze for at least 4-6 hours or until completely solid.

Time of Preparation:

- Approximately 15 minutes (excluding freezing time).

Tips and Tricks:

- Use ripe and sweet berries for a more flavorful popsicle.
- For a textured feel, leave some berry chunks in the mix.
- Run the molds under warm water for easy removal.

Nutritional Value per Serving (1 popsicle):

- Calories: ~120
- Fat: 8g
- Carbohydrates: 10g
- Fiber: 2g
- Protein: 1g

Health Benefits:

- Berries are rich in antioxidants and vitamins.
- Coconut milk provides healthy fats and a creamy texture.

Packaging and Storing:

- Wrap popsicles individually in plastic wrap.
- Store in an airtight container in the freezer for up to 2 months.

Estimated Cost of Preparation:

- $10-$15, depending on the cost of berries and coconut milk.

Precautions:

- Be cautious with popsicle sticks to avoid injury, especially with children.
- Check for any allergies among consumers.

Post-Caution:

- Enjoy these popsicles responsibly as part of a balanced diet.
- Stay hydrated, especially in hot weather.
- Remember to adapt the recipe based on personal preferences and dietary restrictions.

Dark Chocolate Avocado Mousse

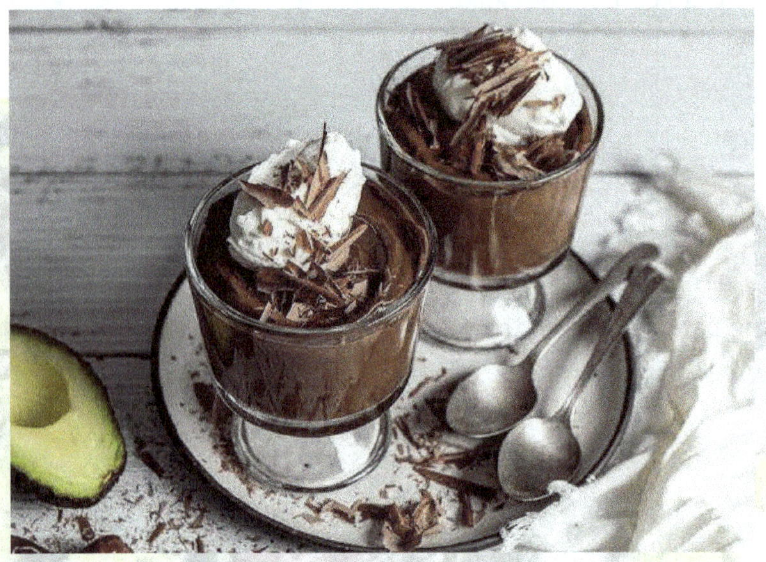

Ingredients:

- 2 ripe avocados, peeled and pitted
- 1/2 cup dark chocolate chips or chopped dark chocolate
- 1/4 cup unsweetened cocoa powder
- 1/4 cup maple syrup or agave syrup
- 1 teaspoon vanilla extract
- Pinch of salt

- Optional toppings: whipped cream, berries, chopped nuts

Procedure:

- Avocado Preparation: In a blender or food processor, combine ripe avocados, cocoa powder, maple syrup, vanilla extract, and a pinch of salt.

- Blend until smooth.

- Chocolate Melting: Melt the dark chocolate using a double boiler or in the microwave in 20-second intervals, stirring in between until smooth.
- Incorporate Chocolate: Add the melted dark chocolate to the avocado mixture.

- Blend again until the mousse is creamy and well combined.

- Chill: Refrigerate the mousse for at least 2 hours to allow it to firm up.

- Approximately 15 minutes (excluding chilling time).

Tips and Tricks:

- Ensure avocados are fully ripe for a smoother texture.
- Adjust sweetness by adding more or less maple syrup based on preference.
- Experiment with different percentages of dark chocolate for varying richness.

Nutritional Value per Serving (1/2 cup):

- Calories: ~200
- Fat: 15g
- Carbohydrates: 20g
- Fiber: 6g
- Protein: 3g

Health Benefits:

- Avocados provide healthy fats and contribute to a creamy texture.
- Dark chocolate contains antioxidants and may have heart health benefits.

Packaging and Storing:

- Divide the mousse into individual serving cups.
- Cover with plastic wrap to prevent oxidation.
- Store in the refrigerator for up to 2 days.

Estimated Cost of Preparation:

- $8-$12, depending on the cost of avocados and dark chocolate.

Precautions:

- Check for any allergies, especially to avocados or dark chocolate.
- Consume in moderation due to the calorie content.

Post-Caution:

- Indulge in this treat mindfully as part of a balanced diet.
- Share the joy of a healthier dessert with friends and family.

Chia Seed Pudding with Mango

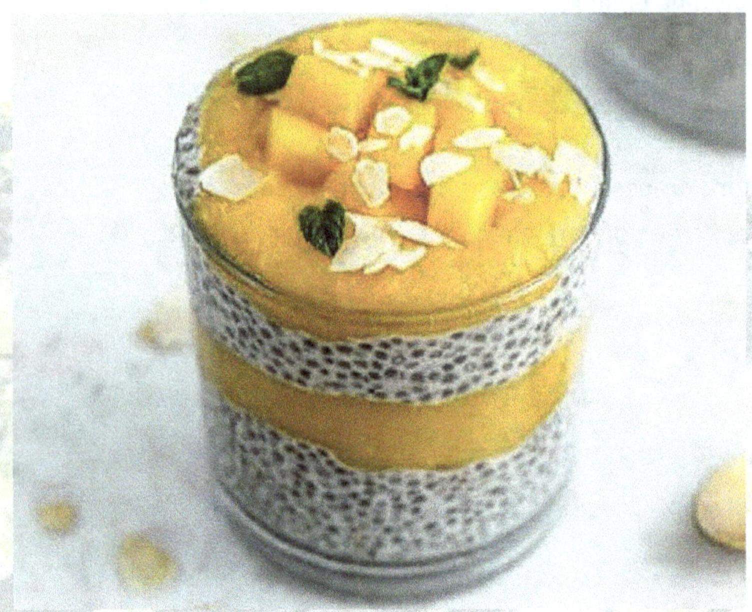

Ingredients:

- 1/4 cup chia seeds
- 1 cup almond milk (or any preferred milk)
- 1 tablespoon honey or maple syrup
- 1/2 teaspoon vanilla extract
- 1 ripe mango, diced

- Optional toppings: sliced almonds, shredded coconut

Procedure:

- Mix Chia Seeds and Liquid: In a bowl, combine chia seeds, almond milk, honey or maple syrup, and vanilla extract.

- Stir well to prevent clumping.

- Refrigerate: Cover the bowl and refrigerate for at least 4 hours or overnight.

- Stir occasionally during the first hour to prevent chia seeds from settling.

- Prepare Mango: Dice the ripe mango into small cubes.
- Assemble: Once the chia pudding has thickened, spoon it into serving glasses or bowls.

- Top with diced mango and any optional toppings.

- 5 minutes for mixing, at least 4 hours for refrigeration.

- Adjust sweetness by varying the amount of honey or maple syrup.
- Experiment with different types of milk for varied flavors.
- Add a pinch of cinnamon for extra warmth.

- Calories: ~200
- Fat: 10g
- Carbohydrates: 25g
- Fiber: 12g
- Protein: 5g

- Chia seeds are rich in omega-3 fatty acids and fiber.
- Mango adds vitamins and antioxidants.

- Portion the chia pudding into individual jars.
- Seal tightly and store in the refrigerator for up to 3 days.

- $5-$8, depending on the cost of chia seeds and mango.

- Ensure chia seeds are well-mixed to avoid clumping.
- Check for allergies, especially to chia seeds or almonds.

- Enjoy this nutritious and delicious pudding as part of a balanced diet.
- Experiment with various fruit toppings for added variety.

CHAPTER 10

BEVERAGES TO BOOST FERTILITY

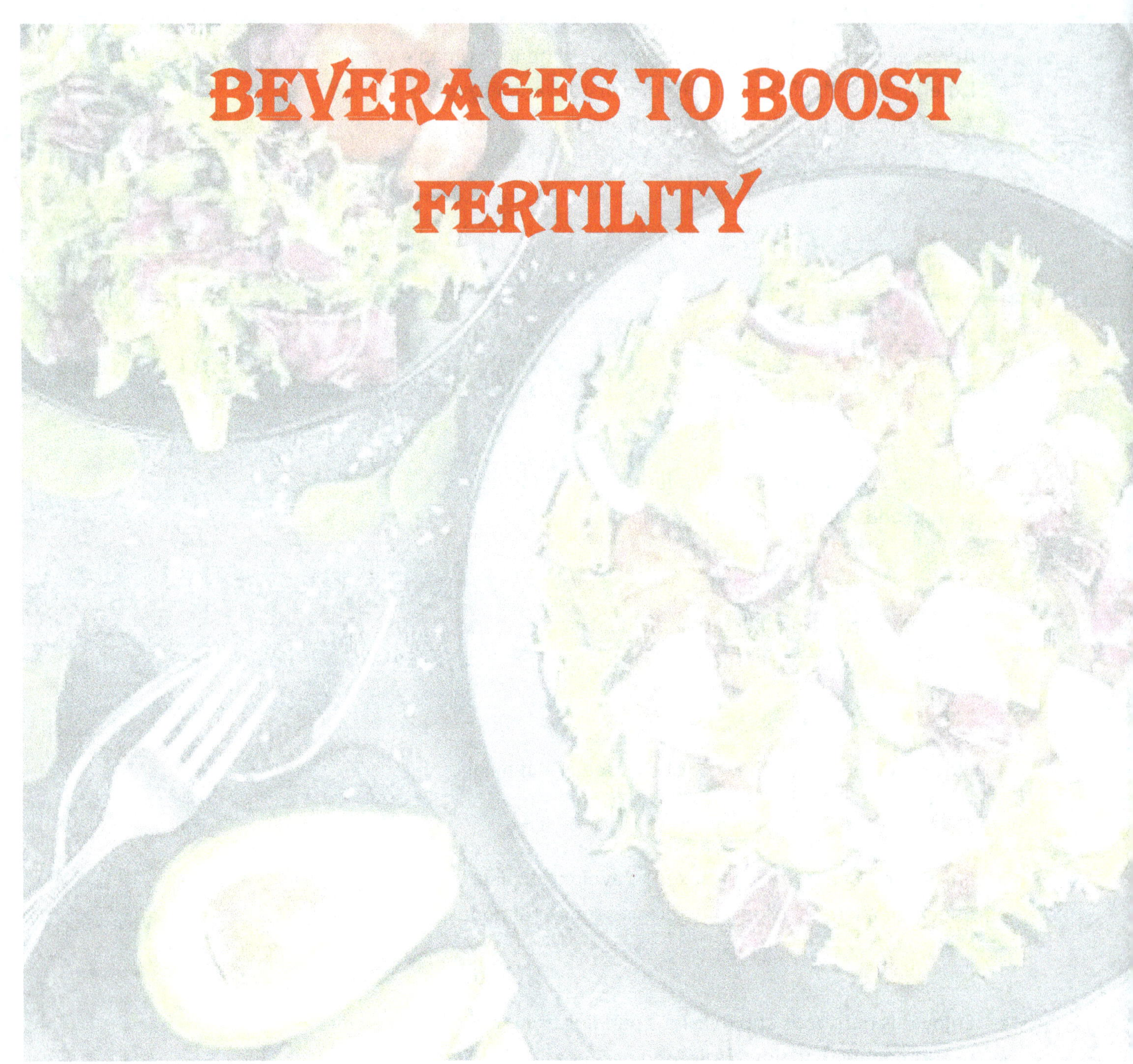

Green Tea Antioxidant Smoothie

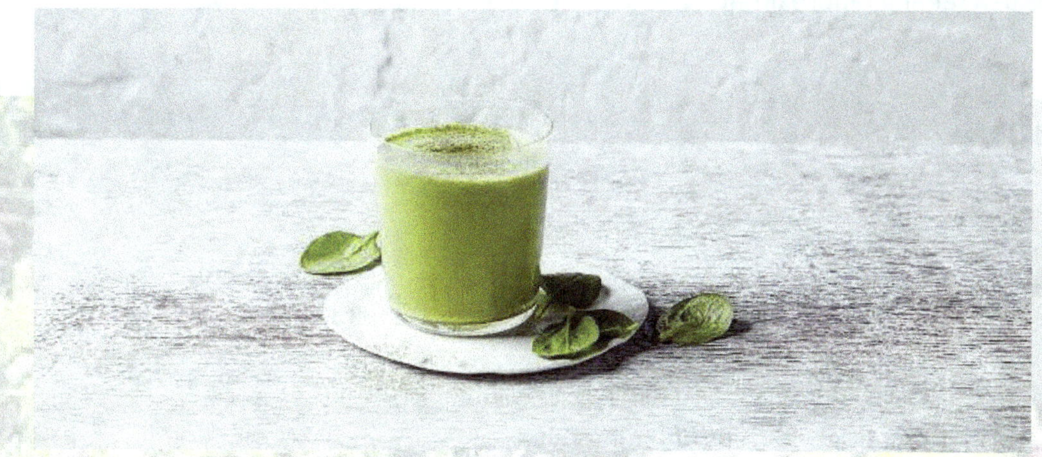

Ingredients:

- 1 cup green tea, brewed and cooled
- 1 frozen banana
- 1/2 cup fresh spinach leaves
- 1/2 cup frozen mixed berries
- 1 tablespoon chia seeds
- 1 tablespoon honey or agave syrup (optional)
- 1/2 cup plain Greek yogurt
- Ice cubes (optional)

Procedure:

- Brew green tea and let it cool to room temperature.
- In a blender, combine cooled green tea, frozen banana, spinach leaves, mixed berries, chia seeds, honey or agave syrup (if using), and Greek yogurt.
- Blend until smooth and creamy.
- Add ice cubes if a colder consistency is desired, and blend again.
- Pour into a glass and serve immediately.

Time of Preparation:

- Approximately 10 minutes.

Tips and Tricks:

- Use frozen fruits for a thicker and creamier texture.
- Adjust sweetness by adding more or less honey/agave according to your preference.

- Experiment with different green tea varieties for unique flavors.

Nutritional Value per Serving (approximate):

- Calories: 180
- Protein: 10g
- Fiber: 7g
- Antioxidants: High content from green tea and berries

Health Benefits:

- Rich in antioxidants, supporting overall health.
- Green tea may boost metabolism and aid in weight management.
- Spinach provides essential vitamins and minerals.
- Chia seeds offer omega-3 fatty acids for heart health.

Packaging and Storing:

- Best consumed fresh, but can be stored in an airtight container in the refrigerator for up to 24 hours.
- Shake well before consuming if refrigerated.

Estimated Cost of Preparation:

- Varies based on location and ingredient brands. Roughly $5-8 per serving.

Precautions:

- Monitor caffeine intake, especially if sensitive.
- Check for allergies to any ingredients.
- Consult a healthcare professional if you have specific dietary concerns.

Post-Caution:

- Enjoy as part of a balanced diet.
- Customize ingredients based on personal preferences or dietary restrictions.
- Share the recipe with others for a healthy treat.

Ginger and Turmeric Infused Water

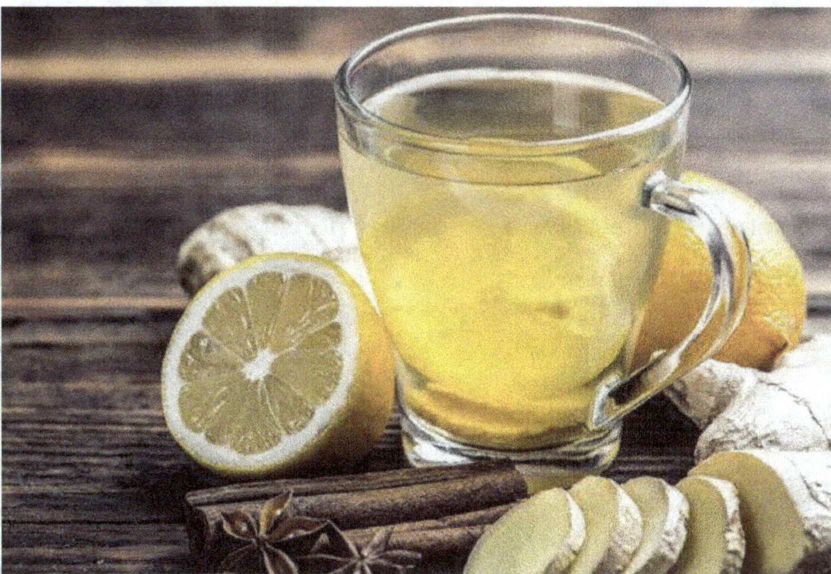

Ingredients:

- 1 small piece of ginger, sliced
- 1 teaspoon turmeric powder or a small turmeric root, sliced
- 1-2 slices of lemon
- 1-2 teaspoons honey (optional)
- 4-5 cups water (filtered or spring water)

Procedure:

- In a pitcher, combine sliced ginger, turmeric, lemon slices, and water.
- Stir well and let it sit for at least 1-2 hours to allow the flavors to infuse.
- Optionally, add honey for sweetness, stirring until it dissolves.
- Strain the mixture to remove ginger, turmeric, and lemon slices.
- Pour the infused water into glasses over ice cubes and enjoy.

Time of Preparation:

- Approximately 5 minutes for preparation, plus 1-2 hours for infusion.

Tips and Tricks:

- Adjust the ginger, turmeric, and lemon quantities based on your taste preferences.
- Experiment with adding other herbs like mint for additional freshness.

- Calories: Negligible
- Ginger and turmeric contribute anti-inflammatory properties.
- Lemon provides vitamin C.

Health Benefits:

- Ginger and turmeric have anti-inflammatory and antioxidant properties.
- May aid digestion and boost immune function.
- Lemon adds a refreshing twist and vitamin C.

Packaging and Storing:

- Store the infused water in the refrigerator for up to 24 hours.
- For on-the-go, use a reusable water bottle.

Estimated Cost of Preparation:

- Varies based on ingredient quality and location. Roughly $2-3 per serving.

Precautions:

- Turmeric may stain surfaces and clothing, handle with care.
- Ginger can be strong; adjust quantity to personal taste.
- Consult with a healthcare professional if you have specific health concerns or conditions.

Post-Caution:

- Incorporate this infused water as part of a balanced diet.
- Stay hydrated and enjoy the refreshing benefits.
- Share the recipe with friends and family for a healthy alternative to sugary drinks.

Fertility-Enhancing Herbal Tea Blend

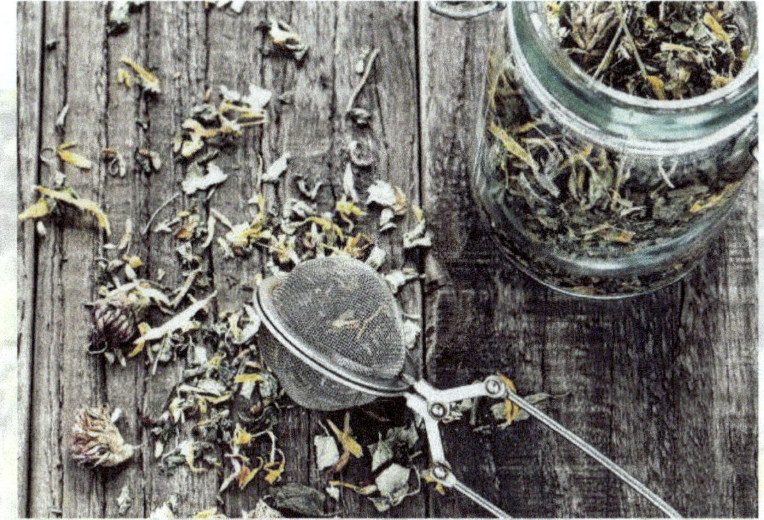

- 1 tablespoon red clover blossoms
- 1 tablespoon nettle leaves
- 1 tablespoon red raspberry leaf
- 1 tablespoon alfalfa leaf
- 1 teaspoon dong quai root
- 1 teaspoon chaste tree berries
- 1 teaspoon licorice root (optional for sweetness)

Procedure:

- In a teapot or infuser, combine all the herbs.
- Boil water and pour it over the herbs.
- Let it steep for 5-7 minutes, or longer for a stronger infusion.
- Strain the tea into a cup and, if desired, add honey for sweetness.
- Enjoy the fertility-enhancing herbal tea warm.

Time of Preparation:

- Approximately 10 minutes.

Tips and Tricks:

- Consult with a healthcare professional before consuming herbal blends, especially during pregnancy.
- Adjust herb quantities based on personal preferences.

- Consume 1-2 cups per day for potential fertility benefits.

Nutritional Value per Serving (approximate):

- Calories: Negligible
- Rich in vitamins and minerals that may support reproductive health.

Health Benefits:

- Red clover and nettle are rich in essential nutrients.
- Red raspberry leaf is believed to support the female reproductive system.
- Dong quai and chaste tree berries are traditionally associated with fertility support.

Packaging and Storing:

- Store the herbal blend in a cool, dark place away from moisture.
- Package in airtight containers to maintain freshness.

Estimated Cost of Preparation:

- Varies based on the quality and source of herbs. Roughly $1-2 per serving.

Precautions:

- Pregnant or nursing individuals should consult a healthcare professional before consuming fertility-enhancing herbs.
- Monitor your body's response and discontinue use if any adverse reactions occur.

Post-Caution:

- This tea is not a guarantee of fertility enhancement; it should be part of a holistic approach.
- Combine with a healthy lifestyle, proper nutrition, and medical advice for comprehensive fertility support.
- Share information responsibly and encourage consultation with healthcare professionals.

Efficient Batch Cooking Strategies For A MTHFR Cookbook Focused On Fertility

Batch cooking tailored to a MTHFR-friendly cookbook for fertility involves thoughtful planning and preparation. The MTHFR gene mutation affects the body's ability to process certain nutrients, emphasizing the need for a nutrient-dense and well-balanced approach. Here are key strategies for efficient batch cooking in this context:

Ingredient Selection:

- Prioritize organic, whole foods rich in methylated nutrients, such as leafy greens, cruciferous vegetables, and lean proteins.
- Choose folate-rich sources like dark leafy greens, broccoli, and lentils as alternatives to synthetic folic acid.

Menu Planning:

- Develop a weekly menu that includes a variety of nutrient-dense meals catering to MTHFR considerations.
- Plan meals that incorporate fertility-boosting ingredients, such as foods rich in omega-3 fatty acids, zinc, and antioxidants.

Batch-Friendly Recipes:

- Select recipes that are easily scalable and adaptable for batch cooking, ensuring consistency in nutrient intake throughout the week.
- Include diverse cooking methods like roasting, steaming, and sautéing to maintain nutritional integrity.

Preparation Efficiency:

- Prep ingredients in bulk, such as chopping vegetables, marinating proteins, and portioning grains, to streamline the cooking process.

- Utilize time-saving kitchen tools like slow cookers, Instant Pots, and sheet pans to maximize efficiency.

- Divide cooked meals into individual or family-sized portions before freezing to facilitate easy reheating.
- Label and date each container to keep track of freshness and optimize meal rotation.

- Incorporate a range of colorful fruits and vegetables to ensure a diverse nutrient profile, promoting overall health and fertility support.
- Experiment with different herbs and spices for flavor enhancement without relying on excessive salt or processed seasonings.

- Incorporate supplements that support MTHFR considerations, such as methylated forms of B-vitamins, into meal planning.
- Coordinate with healthcare professionals to tailor supplementation to individual needs.

- Plan a rotation of meals throughout the week to prevent monotony and ensure a broad spectrum of nutrients.
- Consider creating themed days to simplify planning, such as "Mediterranean Monday" or "Protein-Packed Thursday."
- By combining these strategies, one can efficiently batch cook MTHFR-friendly meals that align with fertility goals, offering both convenience and nutritional optimization. It's essential to consult with a healthcare professional or a nutritionist to personalize the approach based on individual health needs and MTHFR gene considerations.

Stress Management Techniques In The Context Of A MTHFR Cookbook For Fertility

Managing stress is crucial when focusing on fertility, especially for individuals with the MTHFR gene mutation. Chronic stress can negatively impact reproductive health, making it essential to incorporate stress management techniques into a MTHFR-friendly cookbook.

Here's a detailed guide on integrating stress-relief strategies with fertility-focused meal planning:

Mindful Eating Practices:

- Emphasize the importance of mindful eating, encouraging individuals to savor each bite and pay attention to their body's hunger and fullness cues.
- Incorporate relaxation techniques before meals, such as deep breathing or a short meditation, to create a calm environment.

Adaptogenic Herbs and Ingredients:

- Introduce adaptogenic herbs and ingredients into recipes to support the body's response to stress. As an illustration, consider rhodiola, holy basil, and ashwagandha.
- Highlight recipes that incorporate adaptogens in a way that enhances flavor while promoting stress resilience.

Balanced Nutrient Intake:

- Ensure the MTHFR-friendly cookbook includes balanced meals with a focus on nutrients that support the nervous system, such as magnesium, B-vitamins, and omega-3 fatty acids.
- Educate on the importance of maintaining stable blood sugar levels through balanced meals to prevent energy crashes that can contribute to stress.

Hydration and Herbal Teas:

- Encourage regular hydration with water and herbal teas known for their calming properties, such as chamomile or lavender tea.
- Include hydrating recipes, like infused water with cucumber and mint, as well as soothing tea blends in the cookbook.

Meal Prep as a Relaxation Ritual:

- Position meal preparation as a therapeutic activity by creating a calm cooking environment and allowing time for reflection.
- Suggest involving family or a partner in the meal prep process to foster a supportive and social atmosphere.

Incorporate Mood-Boosting Foods:

- Integrate foods that promote the release of serotonin and dopamine, such as dark chocolate, nuts, and seeds, into the cookbook.
- Showcase recipes that use these ingredients in a way that enhances both nutritional and emotional well-being.

Regular Physical Activity:

- Highlight the importance of regular physical activity in stress management and fertility support.
- Suggest recipes with nutrient-dense ingredients that complement an active lifestyle and provide sustained energy.

Mind-Body Techniques:

- Integrate mind-body techniques like yoga, meditation, or progressive muscle relaxation into the stress management approach.
- Recommend specific recipes that align with relaxation practices, such as post-yoga smoothies or meditation-friendly snacks.

Individualized Approach:

- Emphasize the uniqueness of stress management needs and encourage individuals to explore techniques that resonate with them personally.
- Provide resources for additional support, such as stress management workshops or professional counseling services.
- By combining stress management techniques with a MTHFR-friendly cookbook, individuals can optimize their fertility journey by addressing both nutritional and emotional aspects. It's important for individuals to consult with healthcare professionals to create a holistic plan tailored to their specific needs and health conditions.

Exercise And Its Impact On Fertility In The Context Of A MTHFR Cookbook:

Physical activity plays a significant role in fertility, and when considering the MTHFR gene mutation, exercise can be a crucial component in optimizing reproductive health. Incorporating a thoughtful exercise plan alongside a MTHFR-friendly cookbook can enhance overall well-being. Here's a detailed exploration of the connection between exercise and fertility, coupled with dietary recommendations:

Balancing Hormones through Exercise:

- Regular exercise helps balance hormones, including insulin, cortisol, and sex hormones, which is essential for fertility.
- Recommend moderate-intensity activities like brisk walking, cycling, or yoga, promoting hormonal equilibrium without causing excessive stress on the body.

Weight Management:

- Maintain a healthy weight through a combination of exercise and balanced nutrition, as obesity or underweight conditions can impact fertility.
- Include recipes in the MTHFR cookbook that support a balanced and nutrient-dense diet, promoting sustainable weight management.

Enhancing Blood Circulation:

- Exercise improves blood circulation, delivering essential nutrients and oxygen to reproductive organs.
- Emphasize recipes containing foods rich in iron and antioxidants, enhancing the body's ability to transport oxygen and combat oxidative stress.

Stress Reduction:

- Physical activity is a natural stress-reliever, helping to reduce cortisol levels and mitigate the negative impact of stress on fertility.
- Suggest MTHFR-friendly recipes that incorporate stress-reducing nutrients like magnesium and B-vitamins.

Improving Insulin Sensitivity:

- Regular exercise enhances insulin sensitivity, reducing the risk of insulin resistance and supporting metabolic health.

- Feature recipes with low-glycemic index foods that help stabilize blood sugar levels and contribute to improved insulin function.

Fertility-Specific Exercises:

- Introduce exercises that specifically target the pelvic region, such as Kegel exercises and yoga poses, to enhance blood flow to reproductive organs.
- Accompany these exercises with recipes rich in nutrients like zinc and selenium, which are vital for reproductive health.

Promoting Overall Well-being:

- Regular physical activity contributes to overall well-being, improving mood and reducing the risk of conditions that may impact fertility.
- Include recipes with mood-boosting ingredients like omega-3 fatty acids and tryptophan, fostering a positive mental state.

Timing and Intensity:

- Address the importance of balancing exercise intensity and duration to avoid excessive stress on the body, which could negatively impact fertility.
- Suggest meal options in the cookbook that provide sustained energy for different exercise intensities and durations.

Consultation with Healthcare Professionals:

- Encourage individuals to consult with healthcare professionals, including fertility specialists and fitness experts, to tailor exercise plans to their specific needs.
- Stress the importance of personalized advice based on individual health conditions and the MTHFR gene mutation.
- By combining exercise with a MTHFR-friendly cookbook, individuals can create a comprehensive approach to fertility that addresses both nutritional and physical well-being. It is essential for individuals to consult with healthcare professionals to ensure a tailored plan that aligns with their specific health needs and supports their fertility journey.

CONCLUSION

In conclusion, a well-crafted MTHFR Cookbook for Fertility serves as a holistic guide, intertwining the realms of nutrition, stress management, and exercise to empower individuals on their fertility journey. By embracing nutrient-dense recipes tailored to the MTHFR gene mutation, incorporating stress-relief techniques, and promoting mindful exercise, this cookbook offers a comprehensive approach to optimizing reproductive health. Remember, fertility is a multifaceted journey, and consulting with healthcare professionals for personalized guidance ensures a path that aligns with individual needs and the unique considerations associated with the MTHFR gene mutation. May this cookbook not only nourish the body but also inspire confidence and resilience on the path to achieving the dream of building a healthy and happy family.

www.ingramcontent.com/pod-product-compliance
Lightning Source LLC
Chambersburg PA
CBHW080728260726
48660CB00010B/3744